INDEPENDENT
MENTAL HEALTH
ADVOCACY
The Right to Be Heard

INDEPENDENT MENTAL HEALTH ADVOCACY
The Right to Be Heard

Context, Values and Good Practice

Karen Newbigging, Julie Ridley, Mick McKeown, June Sadd,
Karen Machin, Kaaren Cruse, Stephanie De La Haye,
Laura Able and Konstantina Poursanidou

Forewords by Kris Chastey and Toby Brandon

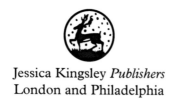

Jessica Kingsley *Publishers*
London and Philadelphia

Boxes 4.1 and 4.3 contains public sector information licensed under the Open Government Licence v3.0. Box 4.4 is reproduced with kind permission of Lucy Costa. Figure 8.3 is reproduced with kind permission of Gateshead Advocacy Information Network. Box 10.1 is reproduced with kind permission of Frank Essery. The bullet list at the end of Chapter 10 with key messages for IMHA providers is reproduced with kind permissino of SCIE. Figure 11.1 is reproduced with kind permission of John Wiley & Sons, Inc. Box 12.3 is reproduced with kind permission of Angela Esslinger. The authors would also like to thank Wayne Lewis, Pete Fleischmann and Rachael Pringle for their kind permission to reproduce material in Chapter 12.

First published in 2015
by Jessica Kingsley Publishers
73 Collier Street
London N1 9BE, UK
and
400 Market Street, Suite 400
Philadelphia, PA 19106, USA

www.jkp.com

Library of Congress Cataloging in Publication Data
A CIP catalog record for this book is available from the Library of Congress.

British Library Cataloguing in Publication Data
A CIP catalogue record for this book is available from the British Library

ISBN 978 1 84905 515 4
eISBN 978 0 85700 930 2

Printed and bound in Great Britain

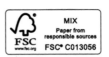

MIX
Paper from
responsible sources
FSC
www.fsc.org   FSC® C013056

This book is dedicated to all of those people who are subject to compulsion and detention under mental health law and who have a right to be heard, which should be upheld by mental health advocacy.

Contents

FOREWORD

KRIS CHASTEY

Being sectioned in hospital is a very lonely, frightening experience. You're desperately hoping and searching for help, information, some clarity over your situation. In my experience of this dark place, it only began to change when along came a light (advocate). I had no idea what an advocate was, let alone how much they could help me. Upon meeting the advocate it became very clear, very quickly, this wasn't just another member of staff. This person listened to me. This person LISTENED. I became a name, a human being again, not just a section. We spoke at length about my situation and how we could go about improving it. The advocate spoke to me like a person, open and honest; nothing was guarded or sugar coated. I asked a question, I got a straight answer. Good or bad, it was the information I was craving. From then on, for every ward round or meeting with the doctor, I'd take the advocate. The advocate asked a question on my behalf, usually getting a positive result or feedback. Me asking that same question, I'd get a 'we'll discuss it as a team and get back to you'; the advocate asked and it's done. Through my time in hospital the advocate became a tool to speed up the process of getting out, asking about my therapy or medication. A good advocate becomes your mouthpiece, asking the questions you need answering, getting you the results you need. My experience of hospital is a place where information doesn't flow to and from the right people. The advocate unblocks this process. By introducing common sense and a dose of reality (in a very unreal situation), you know where you stand; you know what's happening. Working together with my advocate sped up the process of everything I needed, reducing medication, increasing leave, and eventually getting discharged. On many occasions the advocate was unhappy with my situation and wanted answers; answers they got. If I asked those same questions as a patient, at best I wasn't taken seriously, at worst it was seen as a sign that I was becoming unwell. My situation improved the moment I took the chance to get the advocate involved. I took that chance as I figured it couldn't get any worse. I found an ally, a voice of reason, a person who could help me at every step with my journey through hospital. The last step of this was my Tribunal; my advocate sat right next to me, after talking me through the whole process and helping me through it. In hospital, most patients see the advocate as another person to avoid and not trust. They all struggle with the same problems I did: fear, uncertainty and the lack of information that surrounds you in hospital. I found using the advocate was the change that started helping me the most. I saw from my own experience the patients who used the advocate went through the whole hospital process much quicker and seemed much more content with the way things were going. The patients who avoided all contact with the advocate (the majority) struggled through, with all the same problems, unhappy with medication, their leave and their situation. It didn't seem to improve because as a patient on your own, you're not taken seriously or put to the back of the queue. When I took the advocate to ward rounds, the whole weekly meeting became very different. The doctor and the staff became much more efficient, as if just by having the advocate there it kept them on their toes. The dynamic of ward rounds changed; we got answers, clear ideas and a structure on how my care would go. Every question and request was answered and explained there and then. No more 'we'll discuss it as a team and get back to you' – we got a 'yes' or a complete and clear reason for not agreeing. My whole situation was improved by my advocate. I have no doubt of this, but at the same time I'm very aware that the advocate I found was a very GOOD advocate. I know from previous experiences and many stories of other patients this isn't always the case.

Once a week, when the advocate came to the ward, I saw them as the most important person in the building, someone who can get things done. So, from my point of view, the type of people who become advocates is incredibly important. There are many qualities needed to do the job well. I actually consider myself lucky throughout my whole journey through the hospital experience, as I found a very good, helpful advocate, who helped me in my hour of need. I hope every patient finds the advocate they deserve, and they help them in the way I was helped.

Kris Chastey

FOREWORD

TOBY BRANDON

Advocating for advocacy has been a deep interest of mine along with my father David Brandon, who wrote and lectured extensively on it two decades ago. For us advocacy has always been one of those social constructs that is both very simple and very complex. It is simultaneously a straightforward scratched record representation of someone else's interests as if they are your own, whilst also dealing with the complex nuances of powerful organisational structures and professional cultures. Advocacy in essence provides a means to amplify voice and reinforce rights; however, being based in values it becomes very easy for it to be misrepresented and corrupted.

People being detained under the Mental Health Act 1983, amended in 2007, too readily lose their voices and rights alongside their liberty. The current drivers to empower and ensure social justice for these service users are fraught with conflict and contradictions. The application of human rights to mental health is notoriously problematic; historically we can trace the general right to liberty and the requirement for 'due process' back as far as the Magna Carta, now in its 800th year.

I co-authored with Di Barnes a piece of research commissioned in 2002 by the Department of Health into the development of independent specialist advocacy in England and Wales. This work came from the White Paper Reforming the Mental Health Act 2000, which proposed that service users who are subject to the powers of a new Mental Health Act should have access to advocacy. The study found that there was a very positive reaction to the proposals for specialist advocacy, both advocates and service users alike looking forward to a time when individuals have a clear right to access such advocacy services. In the report's findings we reinforced the expectation that these specialist advocacy services should be monitored, evaluated and reviewed by service users themselves. The significance of this book lies in how it has taken this agenda forward through the authenticity of its core commitment to service user co-production within research and writing.

The book stresses that advocacy values are grounded within the recognition of the power disparities between state power enshrined in services and individual freedom of people using services. As part of this the authors also importantly locate advocacy both historically and currently within mental health activism. I would suggest this complements the developing network of recovery colleges, the growth in Mad Studies courses and recent research on shared decision making in mental health care.

The book explores the classic challenges and conflicts inherent in advocacy such as the differences between 'being an advocate' and taking an 'advocacy role', how in terms of rights the Mental Health Act 2007 trumps the earlier Mental Capacity Act 2005, and the dilemmas between the protection and promotion of human rights. In addition the concerns of conceptualising advocacy as a profession and its measurement in terms of both 'soft' and 'hard' outcomes are also usefully examined in detail. Later chapters go on to consider advocacy in terms of values, different cultures, relationships, respect and participation whilst developing a posture born of activism for supporting mental health service users. Much of this presented work can also be linked to issues relating to carers (including family, friends and other supporters).

One significant message from the book is the key importance of respectful relationships in effective, high-quality advocacy provision. This is interestingly aligned to both service user led research and effective care coordination. All three appear to stress relationships built on mutual trust and power sharing, and all require a commitment to co-production.

It has been a pleasure to see the research underpinning this book develop in the last years through numerous conversations and conference presentations. I am unaware of any book that examines mental health advocacy in the same critical detail as this. The work is impressive in its breadth and depth of source material either developed from original research or referred to systematically. I would suggest that it is read in conjunction with the developing work on recovery and other growing frames of wellness. This book clearly presents a sophisticated resource blending mental health history, policy and philosophy. It gives the reader much more than a straightforward exploration of advocacy and provides a multiple perspective examination of how people make sense of mental health. In bringing together direct accounts and experiences of sectioning, restraints and other critical incidents, the authors present a rigorous and creditable body of evidence. This evidence provides a strong platform for future research in the area and should be read by everyone interested in the value of advocacy and in developing both future service provision and mental health theory, including academics, undergraduate and postgraduate students and practitioners, as well as people with lived experience.

Toby Brandon
Reader in Mental Health and Disability
Department of Social Work and Communities
Faculty of Health and Life Sciences
Northumbria University

Acknowledgements

This book has been co-authored and builds on our experience of working together on a Department of Health Policy Research Programme commissioned and funded study of independent mental health advocate services. The views in this book are our own and not necessarily the views of the Department of Health. We have chosen to take a critical look at Independent Mental Health Advocacy (IMHA) to highlight the complexities of this role. We are indebted to Paul Gray, Zemikael Habte-Mariam, Michelle Kiansumba and Doreen Joseph, who worked with us on the original research and have profoundly influenced our thinking. We are very grateful to all those who participated in our original research, particularly those people who we met who were subject to compulsion and whose words we could hear as we wrote. We have included anonymised quotes for illustrative purposes. Finally we would like to thank Lucy Costa, Frank Essery, Angela Esslinger, Pete Fleischmann, Chris Heginbotham, Wayne Lewis, Anne Plumb and Rachael Pringle, for their helpful contributions, and Kate Mercer and Sara Nunes, for their support with the implementation project that has informed our writing.

Abbreviations and acronyms

A4A Action for Advocacy

AIMS Accreditation for Inpatient Mental Health Services

AMHP Approved Mental Health Professional

BAME Black and Asian Minority Ethnic

BNAP British Network for Alternatives to Psychiatry

BSL British Sign Language

CAMHS Child and Adolescent Mental Health Services

CAPO Campaign Against Psychiatric Oppression

CBT Cognitive Behavioural Therapy

CCG Clinical Commissioning Group

CMH Campaign for the Mentally Handicapped

CMHT Community Mental Health Team

CPA Care Programme Approach

CPN Community Psychiatric Nurse

CQC Care Quality Commission

CRPD Convention of the Rights of Persons with Disabilities

CTO Community Treatment Order

DOLS Deprivation of Liberty Safeguards

DRE Delivering Race Equality

DSM *Diagnostic and Statistical Manual*

FOI Freedom of Information request

IAPT Improve Access to Psychological Therapies

ICAS Independent Complaints Advocacy Service

IMCA Independent mental capacity advocacy/advocate

IMHA Independent mental health advocacy/advocate

JSNA Joint Strategic Needs Assessment

LA Local authority

LGBT Lesbian, Gay, Bisexual and Transgender people

MC Act Mental Capacity Act

MDT Multi-disciplinary team

MH Act Mental Health Act

MHSS Mental health system survivors

MHT Mental Health Tribunal

MPU Mental Patients Union

NAG Nottingham Advocacy Group

NAPS National Association of Psychiatric Survivors

NHS National Health Service

NICE National Institute for Health and Care Excellence

NIMHE National Institute for Mental Health in England

NPCSG Nottingham Patients' Council Support Group

PCT Primary Care Trust

PICU Psychiatric Intensive Care Unit

RC Responsible Clinician

SCIE Social Care Institute for Excellence

SPN Social Perspectives Network

SROI Social Return on Investment

SSO Survivors Speak Out

TUPE Transfer of Undertakings Protection of Employment

UKAN United Kingdom Advocacy Network

WHO World Health Organisation

WISH Women in Secure Hospitals, previously known as Women in Special Hospitals

WRAP Wellness Recovery Action Planning

Chapter 1

FROM POWERLESSNESS TO POWER

Introduction

The importance of advocacy has long been recognised by service user movements as a mechanism to achieve social justice and equality and promote rights. Being able to speak for ourselves and to assert our own views, needs and wishes, in other words self-advocacy, is 'the gold standard in being a citizen' (Beresford 2014). This is not always possible, however, and the barriers to self-advocacy include lacking knowledge about rights, lacking confidence or being fearful of the consequences of expressing views. In a mental health context, this is compounded by distress and the difficult and disempowering circumstances of compulsion under the Mental Health Act (MH Act). The power of psychiatry and associated psy-professions, underpinned by a reductive biomedical model, has had a pervasive impact on people's lives and futures, and consequently is a focus for activism in many countries (Russo 2014). This is grounded in social understandings of mental health and recognition that barriers to inclusion and empowerment are social and structural in form, with well-documented associations between socio-economic inequalities and poor mental health evidencing the need for progressive social policies to promote equal citizenship. Collective social action and advocacy, both individual and collective, is also required not only to promote the claims of people experiencing mental health problems but to open up a space for different forms of knowledge, practice and relationships to emerge. In this book, we take a critical look at the value and practice of statutory mental health advocacy, i.e. independent mental health advocate (IMHA) services, its evolution, and its contribution to promoting rights and social justice.

Defining advocacy

Advocacy can be described as the process of identifying with and representing a person's views and concerns, in order to secure enhanced rights and entitlements, undertaken by someone who has little or no conflict of interest. Put more positively, advocacy is rooted in a special, and perhaps unique, relationship between the advocate and the person they support and uses the tools of representation, negotiation and persuasion in order to bring about a beneficial change in the partner's life. Advocacy requires commitment to the 'partner' (person supported by an advocate) but also a determination to see the process through – to aim for something better at the end of the process, either a concrete 'victory' or a greater sense of involvement and empowerment. (Henderson and Pochin 2001, pp.1–2)

Defining advocacy is a complex undertaking. However, the matter of definition is important to consider for a number of reasons, not least because of potential for confusion in light of debates about the role of independent advocacy as opposed to contributions claimed by health and social work professionals (Dalrymple and Boylan 2013; Jugessur and Iles 2009). Furthermore, it is helpful to understand the landscape of advocacy in order to locate the development and practice of IMHA services. Definitions typically frame advocacy as the means for ensuring the voice of the service user is heard (Hugman 1991). Broadly speaking, the service user either speaks for themselves (self-advocacy), or their voice is heard through the intercession of another person. This could be someone who comes to the advocacy role with shared relevant experience (as in peer or collective advocacy), a volunteer who takes on an unpaid advocacy role (citizen advocacy) or is paid to perform the advocacy role (professional advocacy). This version of advocacy resonates with the *Oxford English Dictionary*'s (2nd edition) definition of advocacy as meaning 'to plead or raise one's voice in favour of; to defend or recommend publicly'. Clearly, in a context of diverse advocacy services, neat distinctions are often blurred. Typically, independent advocacy involves a partnership between a concerned member of the community (citizen advocate) or paid professional advocate and a person who may be feeling vulnerable, isolated or disempowered. In these circumstances, the advocate provides support, information and representation to empower the individual (advocacy partner) to express their needs and wishes (Macadam, Watts and Greig 2013; Stewart and MacIntyre 2013).

Mental health advocacy can be a statutory entitlement, such as IMHA services, or provided as a generic service, not just to those detained in hospital or under Community Treatment Orders (CTOs). Those deemed to be lacking capacity who are in the mental health system may also have entitlement to an independent mental capacity advocate (IMCA) under the Mental Capacity Act (MC Act) 2005. Furthermore, some services which assume the title of advocacy are not, in part or wholly, providing advocacy. An example would be a service calling itself advocacy but which in reality provides information and advice or befriending. Simple information giving does not constitute advocacy, yet would be an important element of the process of advocacy if, for instance, there were concerns over a person's awareness of their individual rights. Although not always clear-cut in practice, independent advocacy in mental health takes various forms, and the main types identified from the literature are summarised in Table 1.1.

TABLE 1.1 DIFFERENT FORMS OF ADVOCACY

Type of advocacy	Definition	Development
Self-advocacy	Self-advocacy is about people asserting their own rights, speaking for themselves, expressing their needs and learning to speak for themselves and other people (see Williams, Shoultz and Berglas 1984). This also encompasses concerns about people's rights as citizens, such as their right to meaningful employment (Ward 1998).	Developed in the UK since the 1970s with and by people with learning disabilities, its roots are firmly in the disability movement and related collective action to bring about social change. Now forms an important element of wellness recovery action planning (Jonikas *et al.* 2013).
Collective advocacy (also known as community advocacy)	Collective advocacy involves people speaking up individually or collectively about concerns that affect them. The term community advocacy is more commonly used for collective advocacy to represent the interests of a particular community, for example people from Black and Asian minority ethnic (BAME) communities (Rai-Atkins *et al.* 2002).	Examples include patient councils established within hospitals, active in the UK in the 1980s and 1990s, or alternatively various service user or survivor groupings, autonomously organised in community settings. More latterly, service user involvement forums have multiplied, with different formats reflecting local circumstances, some self-organised, often hosted in the voluntary sector, with others organised in alliance with mental health services and located within them.

cont.

Type of advocacy	Definition	Development
Citizen advocacy (also known as lay advocacy or volunteer advocacy)	An advocacy partnership is set up when an (unpaid) volunteer or ordinary member of the community works with a vulnerable person to ensure their voice is heard in the system, and promotes their point of view in decision making. This partnership is long term.	This form of advocacy was developed in the 1970s in the UK primarily by supporters of normalisation and the principle of having someone involved in the person's life who is not paid to be with them. In this sense, advocacy was seen as part of the process of protecting vulnerable people, ensuring there are people in their lives who care about what happens to them outwith professional roles.
Peer advocacy	Peer advocacy involves people who have 'insider' knowledge as advocates by virtue of sharing the same experience, e.g. age, ethnicity or disability (Harnett 2004).	Similar to the development of self-advocacy and citizen advocacy, and can also be thought of as a form of collective advocacy. Peers are an important strand of recovery-based approaches but may provide a range of support other than advocacy, for example mentoring.
Professional (or paid) advocacy including statutory advocacy	Advocacy is provided by trained and experienced independent advocates and responds to a range of issues. This includes statutory advocacy (IMHAs, IMCAs and Care Act advocates). Professional advocates can work as generic mental health advocates with people at any stage in the mental health service system on short- and long-term issues.	Both IMHAs and IMCAs in England and Wales were introduced under legislation, and it is therefore a right of any eligible person as defined by these Acts to access such statutory forms of advocacy. Care Act advocacy has been more recently introduced in England in relation to adult social care.

Legal advocacy	Based on the principle that lawyers have a responsibility and duty to act for the best interests of their client. It is described as the act of putting an individual's case in the most persuasive manner, establishing people's rights by defending their conduct (Jugessur and Iles 2009).	Under the Mental Health (MH) Act, people who are detained or placed under a CTO have the right to legal representation at Tribunals.
Non-instructed advocacy	Where, for reasons of capacity, individuals are unable to personally instruct their advocate but they may still need an advocate to ensure their rights are upheld. In order to act on the person's behalf, an advocate will spend time observing the advocacy partner, look for ways for the partner to communicate their wishes and, if relevant, gather information from significant others in the partner's life.	Various forms of advocacy can be non-instructed, e.g. citizen advocacy. IMCA is the most widespread form of non-instructed advocacy, since its introduction in 2005.

A further complication is the 'best interests' advocacy role undertaken by health and social work professionals on behalf of their clients/service users/patients, including the conflicts evident for service professionals adopting an advocacy role. Legal advocacy is clearly important in mental health, particularly in respect of compulsion, and we briefly acknowledge this form of advocacy whilst our main focus is on independent (mental health) advocacy. Legal advocacy, however, can have a key role in promoting social change through litigation, law reform and policy development (Stylianos and Kehyayan 2012), and critiquing the basis of mental health law (Perlin and Douard 2008). Many progressive lawyers are also advocates in the campaigning sense, and struggles for civil or human rights in the mental health or disability context are often expressed primarily as appeals to law or legislative reform. Finally, we have not considered advocacy for carers and family members, as IMHA is aimed at people with mental health problems. Nonetheless, carer advocacy forms an important part of the landscape and recognises that carers also have needs and encounter challenges in getting their voice heard by services.

Mental health advocacy and power

Advocacy is grounded in recognition of the power disparities between services and the people using those services (Brandon *et al.* 1995; O'Brien 1987; Silvera and Kapasi 2002), having the intention of mitigating vulnerabilities engendered in such human service systems, promoting change and eliminating barriers to inclusion (Stylianos and Kehyayan 2012). Thus, advocacy has the potential to alter the dynamic within services so that there is greater equality and power sharing, such that the views of individual service users are central to decision making and support their wider citizenship. The impact of this will not only enable someone to reach their personal goals but broaden the range of options available, including alternatives beyond the sphere of professional jurisdiction.

The powerlessness experienced by people with extensive contact with mental health services, and particularly those subject to compulsion, is profound. In many countries the law accords the state powers to detain people with mental health problems in hospital and, in specific circumstances, to treat them, against their will, including in community settings. Legislative compulsion is increasing year on year in the UK and in 2013/14 was at its highest ever recorded annual figure of 53,176 uses of the Act to detain people in hospital for longer than 72 hours (CQC 2015a). Care Quality Commission (CQC) reports of the application of the MH Act in England and Wales continue to make for uncomfortable reading. Despite finding some examples of good practice, significant variations in practice have also been highlighted such that people detained under the MH Act are not always aware of their rights nor routinely involved in decisions about their care and treatment (CQC 2015a), thus leading the CQC to question the extent to which containment and control are being prioritised over the more positive care and treatment aspirations of national mental health policy (CQC 2012, 2015a).

Whether or not the existence of such powers, codified in legislation, constitutes an infringement of human rights is widely debated, particularly by service users (WHO Europe 2014; Wildeman 2013). In such situations, as Kris Chastey describes in his foreword, people can feel extremely disempowered, lonely and bewildered. These experiences of powerlessness include not being understood, being ignored and feeling helpless or insecure (Hooff and Goossensen 2013). Many people can speak out for themselves, but the impact of compulsion, compounded by lack of information, can undermine confidence and self-belief. As Kris describes, advocacy can enable individuals to participate in decisions about their care and treatment and achieve personal goals, and is an essential safeguard to protect rights and facilitate recovery, serving as 'a light in a dark place'.

IMHA services were introduced under reforms to the MH Act 1983 in England and Wales in 2007 as one of a number of safeguards to defend the rights of people subject to compulsion. The incorporation of a statutory right to advocacy into the legal framework for detention and compulsion of people with mental health problems was a relatively unusual innovation, although following a pattern set by both Austria and the Netherlands in the 1990s (Sapey 2013). Its aim was to protect and promote the rights of people subject to compulsion, in a context where other forms of advocacy continued to exist. Its introduction was viewed sceptically by some as a response to the opposition to the MH Act reforms, whilst welcomed by others as a step in the right direction for service user rights (Mental Health Alliance 2008). In this book we explore the role and practice of IMHAs and the opportunities and challenges posed by their introduction. In doing so, we aim to take an appreciative but critical view of IMHA services, locating its development within a broader historical, social and policy context.

Arguably, the coercive and liberty-curtailing nature of much modern psychiatric care is bound up with the application of bio-technologies as part of wider systems of governance (Ingleby 1985; Rose 1990). This is set in a wider context of alleged and actual failings in care and compassion, indicating that the need for an advocacy role within mental health services has never been more pressing (Randall and McKeown 2014). Advocacy generates a potential contribution to empowerment, self-determination and realisation of tangible changes in people's circumstances. Moreover, the very process of advocacy and the advocacy relationship itself can be experienced as a positive and affirming force in people's lives. IMHAs offer possibilities for the views of people detained under the MH Act to be heard and properly considered and for their rights to be upheld. They are, however, situated in difficult territory, in the intersection between the power of the state and individual freedom, between bio-psychosocial hegemony and alternative narratives of distress, and between individual and collective advocacy for social justice for people experiencing mental distress. In this book we consider key questions relating to the role of IMHAs, their purpose, and their position in relation to rights and entitlements. We also debate criticisms of the development of IMHA, as the incorporation of a service user-led initiative into statutory provision.

Overview of the book

This book has been co-written by people with lived experience of mental health problems, and of detention under the MH Act, together with academics in a UK context. This is reflected in different writing styles, which includes personal reflections (Russo and Beresford 2014). We came together on the first large-scale national evaluation of IMHA services in England (Newbigging *et al.* 2012a, 2014), hereafter referred to as 'our study'. This study is the most comprehensive evaluation of IMHA services to date and involved 289 participants in total: 75 people in focus groups and 214 in interviews in selected sites across England. The interviewees included 90 service users with experience of detention in in-patient wards, secure services and on CTOs, as well as IMHAs, carers and mental health professionals (both managers and front-line staff). We have drawn extensively on the findings from this study, further details of which are provided in Chapter 6, and included illustrative quotations from various participants. We have continued to work together in order to translate our findings into practical action and have been involved in efforts to develop resources to promote good practice in the implementation of the duty to provide IMHA services, hereafter referred to as the implementation project (see Useful Resources: SCIE/UCLan 2015).

The chapters in this book are organised into two main parts: the first outlines the context for the development of IMHA services, and the second part examines the practice and experience of IMHA. Each chapter concludes with reflective exercises, a series of questions designed to facilitate individual reflection and dialogue and to support teaching, policy and practice development.

Part 1: Setting the scene

Part 1 locates the recent development of IMHA services in a broader theoretical, historical, legal and practical context as well as exploring the experience of people subject to compulsion. The aim is to enable the reader to develop a critical appreciation of the possibilities and pitfalls of mental health advocacy in the current era. It starts with Chapter 2 and a review of different conceptual frameworks for making sense of mental health problems, exploring key ideas in mental health and recovery. We reflect on the implications of various discourses and critical debates for the practice of mental health advocacy within modern mental health services. We conclude by arguing that advocacy has the potential to democratise the social relations of care and that advocates have a stake in broadening the options available to people in order for them to exercise meaningful choices.

Advocacy is far from being a new concept and, in Chapter 3, we consider the historical development of mental health advocacy services in the UK and its location in associated activism and thinking in the advance of service user/survivor movements. We reflect on the potential tensions that have arisen in the journey of advocacy from the margins to the mainstream.

In Chapter 4, we consider the legal context for advocacy and the contested legislative reform which resulted in the amended MH Act 2007 and the introduction of IMHA services. We briefly explore the interface with other legislation, particularly regarding equalities and human rights, the MC Act 2005 and Deprivation of Liberty Safeguards (DOLS). In considering the legal and ethical context for advocacy, we reflect on the distinction between positive rights (i.e. freedoms for) and negative rights (freedoms from) to explore the conceptualisation of the IMHA role. We hint at some potential tensions, which resonate with the earlier critiques and foreshadow the later discussions regarding challenges in IMHA practice.

In Chapter 5, we explore service users' experiences of detention and compulsion, drawing on first person narratives and research. There are mixed views on the experience of detention, which may reflect methodological problems with some of the studies. We consider the process of detention and compulsion, highlighting issues of power and disempowering effects. This chapter describes how mental health law impacts on people's lives, and the critical role of advocacy in promoting and protecting rights.

To conclude Part 1, we provide an overview of relevant research findings, and comment on the state of the knowledge base for developing IMHA services. We make the case for service users and advocates to become more involved in advocacy research, and conclude with future directions for research focused on advocacy practice and the rights of people subject to compulsion.

Part 2: The practice and experience of independent mental health advocacy services

The second part of this book focuses on the practice and experience of IMHA services from a range of perspectives: service users, advocates, mental health professionals and commissioners. We start with a consideration, in Chapter 7, of the IMHA role and the landscape of IMHA services, including the relationship between IMHA services and other forms of advocacy. In Chapter 8 we focus on the question of what difference the IMHA makes to the lives of advocacy partners and to their care and treatment under the MH Act. Different views on outcomes are explored and we draw the distinction between appreciations of the process of advocacy and a tangible outcome such as being discharged from a section, for example. We provide a summary of potential outcome indicators from a service user perspective, and offer suggestions for routine monitoring and evaluation of advocacy practice. This raises questions about the purpose of IMHA and whether it serves to act as a remedy or merely a palliative to compulsion.

We explore, in Chapter 9, the relevant values, knowledge and skills associated with engaging with advocacy partners and the development of an effective advocacy partnership. This chapter provides a framework for understanding the need for a strong values base (emphasising user-focused practice and a social justice approach), for advocates to be knowledgeable about the mental health law and service system, and to have a skill set that includes good interpersonal skills. These include communication skills with service users; skills for relating and communicating with care provider teams and organisations; and skills in self-management and the organisation of advocacy work. There is a particular focus on the one-to-one advocacy encounter, highlighting relevant issues in the practice of mental health advocacy: engagement; listening; objectivity and independence; and confidentiality and its limits.

A key finding from our study is that those who most needed a voice were least likely to be heard. The focus for Chapter 10 is, therefore, on equalities and the organisation and practice of appropriate advocacy services for diverse communities. Mental health services have a chequered history in their dealings with diversity issues; for example, individuals from minority ethnic groups, women and people identified in relation to their sexuality. We argue that IMHAs can contribute to the process of resolving some of these problems but also need to address equality and diversity issues in their own practice. This will include considering different conceptions of advocacy and the implications for organisational design and delivery.

Chapter 11 explores the role of mental health services in providing a facilitative context for effective IMHA practice and the ways in which staff from different service perspectives (mis)perceive the role of independent advocacy and relevant boundaries. We offer a framework for understanding the dynamics in the relationship between mental health service staff and independent advocates, and the potential impact on IMHA practice. This supports conclusions regarding appropriate staff training to remedy a lack of appreciation of advocacy.

In 2012, with the advent of Clinical Commissioning Groups (CCGs), the responsibility for commissioning IMHA services passed from the National Health Service (NHS) to local authorities (LAs). The way in which commissioning is undertaken and investment in IMHA services have a direct bearing on how they operate and the impact for advocacy partners. In Chapter 12, we look critically at current and ideal commissioning arrangements, and the challenges faced by local authority commissioners. Good practice is discussed, including needs assessments, co-production, service design, resource allocation and monitoring. This chapter concludes by considering good practice in commissioning for high-quality IMHA services, supported by high-quality mental health services and integrated with a range of other forms of advocacy.

A golden thread running through this book is the heritage of advocacy in service user activism, envisioning a different future for people experiencing mental health problems, both individually and collectively. This in turn goes hand in hand with affinities for peer support and service user-led alternatives for care provision. However, the introduction of statutory advocacy has brought with it increasing professionalisation of the role, representing a potential shift away from its activist roots. In the final chapter we explore this paradox, starting with a consideration of the possibilities and prospects for statutory advocacy. We reflect on the emerging debate regarding the professionalisation of advocacy – reviewing the main arguments for and against – proposing that to address these it is necessary to deconstruct, and reconstruct, the very notion of professionalism as it may apply to mental health advocacy. Drawing on the previous chapters, we conclude with reflections on the prospects for the future of IMHA.

A note on terminology

Many of the terms that we have recourse to are widely contested and inadequate in conveying the complexity and rich diversity of people's experience (Wallcraft and Nettle 2009). Furthermore, much of the terminology in common usage has not caught up with current critiques, so we, therefore, reluctantly adopt certain popular terms to reflect their everyday usage, but do so with an appreciation of their problems. We use the terms 'mental distress', 'mental health problems', 'mental disorder' and 'mental illness' somewhat interchangeably to reflect wider usage in specific circumstances or association with particular perspectives. We generally use the term 'service user' to describe people who have experience of using mental health services, although we also refer to 'survivors' in the context of addressing movement politics and particular moments in history.

The term 'service users' in our hands is not intended to negate other identities or to imply that engagement with services is always active and voluntary, as indeed in this context it is not. We have adopted the term 'qualifying patient' to reflect the definition of service users who qualify to use IMHA services, as defined by the MH Act, and in doing so we acknowledge the implicit medicalisation of people's distress. 'Advocacy partner' or 'partner' is used to describe a qualifying patient using IMHA services, and we have adopted this to capture the explicitly egalitarian nature of the advocacy relationship.

We have used the terms 'mental health professional' and 'mental health service staff' interchangeably, and in abbreviated form (staff), to refer to people employed in the delivery of mental health care, as distinct from advocacy.

The term 'carer' is also a source of confusion despite being widely used in official policies and services. We have used the definition from the Carers Trust that:

> A carer is anyone who cares, unpaid, for a friend or family member who due to illness, disability, a mental health problem or an addiction cannot cope without their support. (Carers Trust, 2014)

A full list of abbreviations and acronyms used can be found at the beginning of the book. A glossary is provided at the end.

Part I

SETTING THE SCENE

Chapter 2

UNDERSTANDING THE TERRITORY

Introduction

Arguably, for professional mental health advocates to adequately fulfil their role, a breadth of understanding of key concepts and theories of mental health and 'illness' (effectively, knowledge of how different people and personnel make sense of mental distress) is warranted for a number of reasons:

- to be able to reflect critically on competing theories of the nature of mental health and 'illness', as well as appraise the respective merits and limitations of these various theoretical perspectives, bolstering the advocate's capability to engage in debate and discussion with clinicians and health professionals

- to be aware of the extent that controversy and consensus within and between various theories of mental distress can open up possibilities to challenge dogmatic prescriptions for care and treatment and exploration of alternatives in support of individuals wishing to exercise choice (a policy rhetoric of choice is often promulgated against a backdrop of sparse meaningful alternatives within services)

- to become more familiar with and recognise the language associated with exposition of, or allegiance to, specific theories

- to judge which perspectives are more likely to inform service provision and why;

and most importantly:

- to enable advocates to credibly and confidently engage in dialogue with care team practitioners and mental health service users.

We contend that none of the above suggests an abrogation of the advocacy mission to be an objective, dispassionate supporter of service user voice. Rather, the desirability of awareness of different ways of making sense of mental distress is intimately bound up with an appreciation that such knowledge can be significantly 'loaded' and is often indivisible from the exercise of power. The fact that this knowledge/power is often in the hands of practitioners who hold to a fairly narrow episteme of biological psychiatry arguably goes to the heart of concerns over compulsion, coercion, rights and liberties. After all, it is such matters that more often than not precipitate the involvement of an advocate in the first place.

Accounting for mental health and 'illness'

The concept of mental health, and its corollary 'mental illness', are controversial subjects in the domains of human inquiry and the practice of welfare services. A variety of theoretical perspectives and competing explanations span this contested territory, generating continuing critical debate over these complex issues. To a greater or lesser degree these debates inform the practice of mental health services as well as criticism of them. Similarly, different individuals, whether care team staff, service users or advocates, will have their own subjective affinities for particular ways of making sense of mental health and 'illness'. In this chapter, there is no intention to favour one account of mental health or 'illness' over another. What we are interested in here is to enable mental health advocates to critically appraise the various accounts against each other, and develop an awareness of their role in informing mental health care practice. It is important to remember that none of the different perspectives has an absolute claim to know the 'truth' about what mental health or mental distress is, or the latter's possible cause. Particular theories for making sense of mental health and distress are typically associated with different forms of care and treatment, though it is worth noting that many of the alternatives are not necessarily freely or routinely available across mental health services.

In a selective appraisal of different perspectives on mental health and 'illness' we will look in turn at:

- psychiatric accounts

- psychological accounts

- sociological accounts

- lay and mental health service user/survivor accounts.

We will also discuss developments which may indicate how critical perspectives on mental health and 'illness' have influenced a shift towards more inclusive and pluralistic practices, based on notions of recovery and 'therapeutic alliances'.

Psychiatric accounts

We turn first to psychiatric accounts, not because we wish to privilege these above others, but rather to acknowledge their organising power within modern mental health care services within which advocates must operate. Psychiatrists are the dominant group in such services, reflecting the hegemony of medicine across all health care and the broader post-enlightenment ascendancy of scientific ideas. They have also, arguably, operated an opportunistic professionalisation trajectory, benefiting from governance imperatives concerned with the containment of risk (Rose 1990). These socio-historical developments consolidating medical interests have been supported by a trinity of government, the law and globalising businesses. Not least in all of this has been the role of *Big Pharma* and its marketing through the media in strengthening the influence of the biomedical model and psychiatry (Bentall 2009; Moncrieff 2003, 2006, 2009, 2013).

According to a reductionist, simplistic version of the medical model, health problems are explained in terms of disease or illness. Specific illnesses are recognised and diagnosed by their indicative signs and symptoms, and are remedied by employment of the appropriate cure, usually involving some form of medication or physical intervention. From this perspective, the state of illness is discontinuous with a state of wellness: that is, normality and abnormality (pathology) are clearly distinguishable.

For biomedical psychiatry, mental 'illnesses' arise because of problems in brain functioning and are, hence, treatable by focusing on the brain. Typically, this involves attempts to remediate supposed discrepancies in brain biochemistry by the administration of psychotropic medication. Because of the complexities of the brain compared to other organs there is a large amount of uncertainty and imprecision regarding the role of specific brain structures and neurotransmitters in the cause and course of 'mental disorder' (Kendell 1993). It has been argued that the employment of powerful imaging technologies in increasingly sophisticated neuroscientific research, as well as biogenetic research, promise to offer new insights into the relationship between mental activity/states and the structure and functioning of the brain, and the relationship between genetic factors and 'mental disorders' alike (Bullmore, Fletcher and Jones 2009). It is worth noting that the first author of the latter paper is a part-time employee and shareholder in GlaxoSmithKline.

Reduced to its most simple terms, the psychiatric account focuses on biological, physiological and genetic factors. Because the explanations for mental health problems are grounded in physicality, the body rather than the mind, the treatments are, likewise, physical. In simple terms, the biomedical process of diagnosis and treatment is dependent upon acceptance by individuals of the validity of the psychiatric explanation for their problems, usually referred to as 'insight', leading to compliance with the prescribed pharmacological or physical treatment. Such notions of unrefracted compliance are complicated for many by the overlay of compulsion and coercion within the system, with many service users effectively compelled to comply directly, or the possibility of compulsion indirectly playing into decisions to take medication. Another significant factor for service user choice in this arena is the relative absence of readymade or freely available alternatives to treatment by medication.

Despite undoubted complexities surrounding issues of medication concordance in particular, such a diagnostic and treatment process requires only a passive role on behalf of the patient. At a quite fundamental level, this makes the case for advocacy support, and it is not surprising that many requests for advocacy are framed around issues of voice and choice within the prescribing process.

Most modern psychiatrists, however, would reject such a reductionist view of mental health difficulties and of their own practice. Contemporary practice has moved to incorporate a much more eclectic range of treatment options, including social and psychological therapies, and a conceptual framework which includes a complex of explanatory factors. Hence, a bio-psychosocial model which recognises the complex interplay of social, psychological and biological factors in making sense of mental health problems has been gaining ground in the arena of mental health (Double 2007; Kendell 2001). Latterly this has evolved into the policy and practices of recovery and co-production (Deegan 1994; Perkins and Slade 2012; Shepherd, Boardman and Slade 2007; Slay and Stephens 2013). Despite some undoubted progress in this vein, the bio-psychosocial model has been roundly criticised as lacking a persuasive theoretical basis (Ghaemi 2009; McLaren 1998; Pilgrim 2002; Read, Bentall and Fosse 2014) and, similarly, the recovery paradigm for departing from survivor activism roots towards co-option under psychiatry (Harper and Speed 2014; Mental Health Recovery Study Working Group 2009).

More critical accounts have de-emphasised the supposed biological basis for mental distress and striven to foreground social factors in causation and social-relational caring responses. For example, the Critical Psychiatry Network in the UK has persuasively argued for a range of alternatives to simple bio-psychiatry (Thomas 2014). Likewise, authors such as Joanna Moncrieff (2009) and Robert Whittaker (2002, 2010) have contributed to a trenchant critique of the scientific basis of psychopharmacology and prescribing practices. This criticism does not necessarily discount the importance of the brain sciences and psychopharmacology. Rather, it is convincingly argued that psychiatry needs to move beyond the dominance of its current, technological knowledge paradigm and begin to 'position the ethical and hermeneutic aspects of psychiatrists' work as primary, thereby highlighting the importance of examining values, relationships, politics and the ethical basis of care and caring' (Bracken *et al.* 2012, p.432).

Various commentators have drawn attention to deficiencies in biomedical models of 'mental illness', specifically:

- lack of attention to social and structural aspects/ determinants of mental distress including child abuse and other forms of violence and trauma (Bentall 2009; Read *et al.* 2014)

- over-emphasis on individual, internal, biological and genetic aspects of 'mental illness' (Cromby and Bell 2015; Luchins 2004)

- problems surrounding the categorical approach to diagnosis associated with *The Diagnostic and Statistical Manual* (DSM) and promoting rigid and narrow perceptions of what is 'normal' (Bentall 2013; Kinderman *et al.* 2013; Pilgrim 2014a)

- dismissal of individuals' own frameworks and understandings of their experiences of mental distress, resulting in forms of 'epistemic/testimonial injustice' (Carel and Kidd 2014; Fricker 2007) and 'epistemic violence' (Liegghio 2013).

The emergence of more complex explanatory frameworks and models of practice in mental health to counteract biomedical psychiatric reductionism can be viewed in conjunction with broader problems of modernity, constituting what has been described as 'a legitimacy crisis' for psychiatry (Grob 2011; Lafrance and McKenzie-Mohr 2013; Pilgrim 2012a, 2014b; Rosenburg 1975). Consequently, Bracken and Thomas (2005) have posited a post-psychiatry for a post-modern world.

Interestingly, Simon Wessely (2014, p.1), current President of the Royal College of Psychiatrists, refutes claims that psychiatry is in the midst of a watershed moment and remarks '*The real crisis in psychiatry is that there isn't enough of it.*'

Usually, when the psychiatric account is criticised, it is the reductionist, simplistic version of the medical model which is found fault with. But, if the theory and practice of psychiatry is more sophisticated, then critical engagement with it may have to be tempered and more appropriately targeted. Various contributions from psychology and sociology either complement trends in contemporary psychiatry or furnish continuing critical debate. These contributions are addressed below.

Psychological accounts

There are various perspectives within psychology which inform different understandings of the nature of mental health problems and suggest different treatment interventions. Classically, the focus for interventions is on the individual, though social psychological accounts and systemic therapies are concerned foremost with social networks and groups. Put simply, the psychology of individuals can be theorised as comprising the study of three interlinked domains:

- emotions

- cognitions

- behaviour.

The different conceptual frameworks and interventions within psychology can be seen as roughly corresponding to these three areas. In the analysis that follows, psychodynamic, cognitive, behavioural and cognitive behavioural theories and therapies are briefly discussed. Humanistic theories and therapies are also considered that in one sense reflect an attempt to integrate aspects of all three domains of emotion, cognition and behaviour.

PSYCHODYNAMIC THEORIES AND THERAPIES

Psychodynamic therapies are grounded in the work of Sigmund Freud and his many disciples and dissenters. Despite this territory constituting an eclectic breadth of approaches and theories, there are various common strands. Mental health problems are described and defined in terms of psychopathology, which arises in the dynamic interplay between the conscious and unconscious mind. Such problems are felt to be caused by adverse emotional experiences, especially those forged in childhood, which disrupt normal patterns of psychosexual development. Psychodynamic therapies are classically typified in the long-term relationship between an individual and the therapist, aimed at uncovering important events and associated emotions from the unconscious mind. Group analysis techniques supported the historical development of therapeutic communities which, at their best, represent a democratisation of the relationships of mental health care and open up possibilities for expression of service user voice and peer support. Spandler (2006) has argued that in some instances the evening out of power relations at stake in therapeutic communities was opportune in facilitating service user and staff alliances to the benefit of a critical survivor movement. This was arguably the case in the emergence of the Mental Patients Union (MPU) at Paddington Day Hospital in the 1970s, associated with an industrial dispute to defend the service. Yet the MPU was also able to organise in the seemingly less propitious environs of the asylums (Survivors History Group 2012).

BEHAVIOURAL THEORIES AND THERAPIES

In its early days, academic psychology was characterised by the dominance of the behavioural school, which was linked to the efforts of the discipline to establish an 'objective', scientific basis for itself. As such, reflection on the internal world of individuals was rejected as so much subjective introspection. Rather, the focus was shifted away from the immeasurable psyche to what was viewed as the objectively quantifiable domain of behaviour. Theoretically, human development was seen in terms of the learning of a repertoire of adaptive or maladaptive behaviours. Put simply, such learning would proceed on the basis of reinforcing desired behaviours through a process of reward and punishment. Examples of behavioural treatment approaches include systematic desensitisation for phobias or the token economy approach to modifying behaviour in institutional settings.

COGNITIVE AND COGNITIVE BEHAVIOURAL THEORIES AND THERAPIES

To some extent, increased availability of 'talking treatments' has long been called for by service users/survivors (Rogers, Pilgrim and Lacey 1993). The most fashionable psychological approaches in modern UK mental health services tend to be cognitive or cognitive behavioural interventions; they are often labelled CBT (cognitive behavioural therapy) and have formed the cornerstone of recent initiatives to improve access to psychological therapies (IAPT). The relative prevalence of CBT within UK mental health services has been linked to government interest in supposed links between the economy, productivity and mental well-being (Layard 2013; Pilgrim 2008a). This has been reinforced by the adoption of CBT by National Institute for Health and Care Excellence (NICE) guidelines and the fact that they tend, on the whole, to be brief and, hence, a lot less costly than long-term psychodynamic psychotherapies, for example.

These therapies were developed largely to treat problems of mood, such as anxiety or depression, but have more recently been applied to helping people who are disturbed by hearing voices or having distressing thoughts. This latter group would usually attract a diagnosis of serious 'mental illness', such as 'schizophrenia' or 'bi-polar disorder'. A range of approaches used with this client group have now been evaluated which include CBT and family therapy and are usually described in services as psychosocial interventions (Mueser *et al.* 2013). The potential contribution that has been shown to be made by psychosocial interventions in this context has been something of a breakthrough, as such interventions represent the first non-pharmaceutical approaches to be found to be helpful for people with a diagnosis of serious 'mental illness' (Morrison *et al.* 2014).

The CBT model reflects an approach to understanding the relationship between thoughts, emotions and behaviour, regardless of whether they are considered 'functional/adaptive' or 'dysfunctional/maladaptive', which enables therapists to adopt a normalising philosophy towards clients and their experiences. Thus, the range of possible experiences are seen as existing on a continuum, rather than necessarily being separable into categories indicating 'normality' and 'abnormality'.

HUMANISTIC THEORIES AND THERAPIES

Humanistic therapies are geared towards helping people to achieve an integration of all aspects of their self: conscious dimensions such as thoughts, feelings and actions, and unconscious elements such as dreams. It has been argued that humanistic psychology has the least well-articulated research base, yet many of its concepts are extremely well known, embedded in the training of practitioners such as nurses, and, even if poorly understood, are flexibly demonstrated in the best relational care (Benjamin 2011). For example, the work of Carl Rogers, John Heron and Hildegard Peplau has been widely taught in the professional training of mental health personnel (Ashmore and Banks 2004; Purdy 1997; Williams and Stickley 2010). In this work, people are viewed as inherently creative and motivated towards personal growth and development and realisation of their potential, with self-actualisation being the ultimate goal. To some extent, the recent vogue for positive psychology is grounded in humanistic principles (Robbins 2008).

Humanistic therapies are typically non-directive, working to assist people to resolve their own problems, and are exemplified in Rogers' person-centred counselling (Rogers 1967). This approach suggests three core conditions for personal growth, which the counsellor endeavours to facilitate in the therapeutic encounter. The Rogerian core conditions are:

- non-judgmental positive regard

- empathic responding

- genuineness.

In Rogers' person-centred counselling, advice giving is avoided. The therapist aims to present as a warm and caring person, encouraging the development of self-respect and confidence in the client so that they are enabled to more effectively resolve their problems.

Sociological accounts

The key theoretical alternatives to the clinical domains of psychiatry and psychology are offered by sociological accounts. Simply speaking, sociology attempts to understand the behaviour of individuals or collective groups in 'social' terms. Anne Rogers and David Pilgrim (2014) describe a number of theoretical perspectives within their comprehensive *Sociology of Mental Health and Illness*:

- social causation

- social reaction and labelling

- hermeneutics

- social constructivism

- social realism.

Most of these sub-disciplines of sociology as applied to mental health are not completely independent of each other. Social causation theories are broadly accepting of psychiatric diagnostic categories, and look to account for the extent or severity of mental disorder in terms of social factors, typically environmental or psychosocial stress. Labelling theory argues that the sort of behaviour that would attract a psychiatric diagnosis is actually amplified by the attachment of the label. Hermeneutics are concerned with interpretations of the world and human interaction; phenomenology, for example, holds that all people are perpetually engaged in making sense of their world and that these understandings and exchanges of meaning can be studied. The symbolic interactionist school and the work of Goffman on

Asylums (1961) and *Stigma* (1963) are examples of this broad approach.

Social constructivist theorising, sometimes referred to as post-structural or post-modern, has been hugely influenced by the work of Michel Foucault (1965). Such accounts of mental health have stressed the social control functions of mental health services, within a so-called psy-complex (Ingleby 1985; Rose 1990), and highlight the negative effect of constructions of difference and self–other distinctions (Crowe 2000). This critique connects with theorising about the 'colonial' features of the psychiatric enterprise, which is broader than, but includes, particular forms of racism (Fanon 1952/2008; Foucault 2003; Penson 2014; Sadd 2014).

Critical realist accounts are favoured by Rogers and Pilgrim (2014, p.13), who locate such ideas thus:

> Social realists consider that human action is neither mechanistically determined by social reality nor does intentionality (voluntary human action) simply construct social reality. Instead, society exists prior to the lives of people but they become agents who reproduce or transform that society.

This approach is comfortable with considering a complex interaction of different social, economic and political influences upon mental health, and as such is, on the face of it, compatible with the aforementioned bio-psychosocial model. However, most critical realists object to the way in which that model appears in practice to be too uncritical of foundational medical constructs (Pilgrim 2013).

Of course, the various sociological and psychological accounts can overlap. Society is made up of individuals, and macro-social forces are always evident in interaction with individual agency and motivations. This is recognised in branches of social psychology and, indeed, social psychiatry. Arguably, in the 1950s, psychiatry as a discipline was on a much more social tack and, at this time, the World Health Organization (WHO) was able to proclaim:

> The most important single long-term principle for the
> future work of WHO in the fostering of mental health is the
> encouragement of the incorporation into public health work
> of the responsibility for promoting the mental as well as the
> physical health of the community. (WHO 1958)

This positioning was associated with interest in relational
and democratising dimensions of therapeutic communities,
and it lives on in a somewhat denuded form in the Enabling
Environments initiative sponsored by the Royal College of
Psychiatrists (Johnson and Haigh 2011). Human geographers
such as Parr (2000) have also persuasively theorised on the
importance of place and space for mental health and influencing
personal agency within different care settings. Left-leaning
theorists working within critical social theory perspectives,
such as the Frankfurt School scholars Erich Fromm (see 1956)
and Herbert Marcuse (see 1964), for instance, can be seen to
have established a psychosocial synthesis of psychodynamic
psychological ideas and sociological theory.

PUBLIC PERSPECTIVES ON MENTAL HEALTH

Rogers and Pilgrim (2014; first published 1999) make the point
that a notion of disturbed emotions or behaviour described as
'madness' is common across all cultures. They also make the point
that a notion of 'madness' is often associated with negative public
attitudes towards the mentally unwell, typically associated with
almost atavistic fears (Evans-Lacko, Henderson and Thornicroft
2013). The most obvious example of this is the belief that people
with a mental 'illness' are more likely to be dangerous or violent
and unpredictable. Philo and colleagues from the Glasgow
University Media Group (1996) studied the interplay between
media representations of 'madness' and attitudes held by the
general public. This research found that public attitudes towards
'mental illness' did not operate entirely like attitudes in other
contexts. Usually, the influence of the media would be seen to
be important in reinforcing views one already held, but relatively
ineffective in changing previously held opinions. Contrary to
all other studies of media influence to date, the fear of violence

linked to 'mental illness' was unlikely to be counteracted by personal positive experiences of individual people with 'mental illness' who were not violent. In previous studies of public attitudes towards striking refuse collectors, for instance, if the research subject actually knew a striker, they would disbelieve sensationalist stories in the press.

Lay and mental health service user/survivor accounts

Importantly, the contested territory of understandings of mental health has been hugely contributed to by discourses provided by mental health service users and survivors themselves. Such accounts include attempts at describing and understanding the personal experience of mental health problems and views on the quality and appropriateness of mental health services. It is essential to bear in mind that mental health service user and survivor perspectives do not constitute an homogeneous set of ideas. Examples of note include those sets of service user/survivor views which have been influential in attempts to normalise the range of experiences of individuals and associated self-help initiatives. In some instances, these views have coincided with or influenced practice and service developments in the mental health arena. An example of this is the attention paid to personal life history and coping strategies within psychosocial interventions and the influence of the 'Hearing Voices Network' on such practice and independently (Romme and Escher 1993).

Furthermore, critical service user/survivor perspectives on mental health and 'illness' have influenced mental health policy and shaped important policy shifts – for example, the emergence of Patient/Service User and Public Involvement in mental health research as a key policy driver in the UK in the last decade and positive contributions to practitioner training (Beresford 2002a; McKeown and Jones 2014; Sweeney et al. 2009).

The growth of such mental health service user/survivor influences has been explained in terms of social movement theories (Rogers and Pilgrim 1991). The notion of 'a new social movement' has been attached to less formally organised campaigning and protest groups in order to distinguish them from older groupings such as the trade unions or other mass membership organisations, which were arguably bogged down in bureaucracy, increasingly incorporated into the establishment, and hence less likely to pursue radical change. Various contemporary and historical examples of health and welfare movements have included, or singularly organised, the voice of service user or survivor activists. Notable historical examples include Survivors Speak Out and the MPU (see Chapter 3) and, currently in these times of austerity, budget cuts and politicised antipathy to welfare benefits, alliances have been formed within which survivor activists are prominent. These include groups such as Disabled People Against the Cuts and Black Triangle (Scott 2014).

In the context of mental health politics, an interesting example of a campaigning and protest group is 'Mad Pride'. Mad Pride might be understood to have two functions. The first, internal function is to draw people with experiences of mental distress together and get them to take a positive view of their situation in order to set about achieving greater civil liberties for people with mental health problems. By celebrating diversity, attitudes can be changed. By belonging to a group, people who before were isolated can find a new strength. The second function is external: to change perceptions of mental health issues with the wider public. In particular, Mad Pride and other movement groups campaign against forced treatment and to widen access to alternative and holistic care. Mad Pride mirrors groups such as Gay Pride in encouraging openness about surviving the mental health system, and reclaiming previously stigmatising language (Shaughnessy 2001). Interestingly, official anti-stigma campaigns are not immune from this critique, as they arguably consolidate the biomedical frame with claims that 'mental illness is an illness just like any other illness' (Pilgrim and Rogers 2005).

Internationally, these concerns have been taken up within the emergent field of Mad Studies, a critically engaged wing of disability studies (Burstow, LeFrançois and Diamond 2014; LeFrançois, Menzies and Reaume 2014; Russo and Beresford 2014). Critical scholars and service user allies have reappraised 'biomedicalism and psychiatrisation' to develop the notion of 'sanism' as a distinct form of prejudice and source of discrimination. As such, acts of diagnosis and the associated labels of 'mental illness' themselves constitute *sanism* and *sanist* discourse and practices (Burstow and LeFrançois 2014).

Alternative forms of care for mental distress

The various critical accounts of mental health and the quality and nature of psychiatric care have led to consideration and implementation of different approaches to service provision and independent living. Some of these initiatives have been user-led alternatives, grounded in survivor movement campaigning, such as crisis houses for instance (Pinfold 2000; Wallcraft *et al.* 2011). Others have been established by critically minded practitioners, often in alliance with radical service users.

Campaigning service users and survivors have been in the vanguard of arguing for the replacement of simple bio-medicine with a social model of mental health that could shape more supportive services and frame legislation (Beresford 2002b, 2005; Beresford, Nettle and Perring 2010). This campaigning has been sustained by the Social Perspectives Network (SPN) (SPN 2002) and there have been associated efforts to cascade this thinking into practitioner education (Tew 2002). Further critique has troubled the social model of disability and urged caution in any attempt to apply it too simplistically to mental health or distress (Spandler, Anderson and Sapey 2015). Not unconnectedly, others have argued for initiatives that build upon community strengths, assets and solidarity, developing communities and empowering them in relation to statutory services (Thomas 2014). Aspects of urban life in particular can be detrimental to people's mental health, but resilience and cooperation can be deepened in communities to the benefit of everybody's well-being; in this sense we can promote prosocial places.[1]

---

1   See the Prosocial Place Programme (https://sites.google.com/site/prosocialplace/home).

Inspired by external critique, such as that furnished by the Hearing Voices movement, and evidence supporting the key role of trauma in the course of mental ill health, critical strands within clinical psychology have developed practices that locate aspects of mental distress that would ordinarily attract a psychiatric diagnosis on a continuum of human experience. Subsequent interventions focus upon self-identified complaints rather than implicit biology or bio-chemistry and emphasise psychological therapies and the simple value of talking about one's experiences (Bentall 2009; Cooke 2014). Novel approaches to 'therapeutic alliances' between mental health service users and mental health professionals are grounded in an acknowledgement of, and respect for, individuals' own personal constructs of their experiences and problems as the starting point for collaborative efforts towards problem resolution or improving quality of life. Such approaches to working alliances between service users and mental health professionals are exemplified internationally by alternative models of support for people in crisis such as Open Dialogue (Seikkula and Olson 2003), Healing Homes (Mackler 2014) and Soteria (Bola and Mosher 2003; Calton *et al.* 2008; Mosher 1999), models which have originated in Finland/Lapland, Sweden and the USA respectively.

These latter approaches to service provision are framed in terms of relational aspects of care, emphasising high-quality communication or dialogic interaction, and can be delivered as alternatives to medication or in a minimal medication context. There has also been a recent growth of interest in support for service users to come off medication safely, ideally avoiding harmful rebound effects (Aldridge 2012; Hall 2012; Thomas 2014).

As such, all of these alternatives to mainstream care and treatment are representative of wider efforts to democratise the social relations of care for those in mental distress. Interestingly, it can be argued that such spaces, whereby the democratic voice of service recipients is respected and attended to, are at the heart of advocacy practice. At the very least, practising advocates have an interest in the possible expansion of care and treatment alternatives if service users, wherever they are situated, are to be able to exercise meaningful choices.

Conclusions

In conclusion, it is worth stressing the importance of and implications for advocates being aware of the existence of competing understandings of mental health and distress and the different associated possibilities for service configuration. Given the association of biological psychiatry with compulsion and coercion, arguably it is imperative for independent mental health advocates to develop appreciation and knowledge of mental health and 'illness'. Critical understanding is necessary to support autonomous self-determination on the part of advocacy partners and to fulfil a more systemic advocacy role of challenging injustice and the negative impact of the exercise of psychiatric power. Some argue that advocates may not need to admit such understandings to adequately perform their role, but ultimately we disagree. This is justified not least because advocacy can be seen to have historical roots in survivor movement politics and activism.

One such activist, Peter Sedgwick (1982, p.256), remarked that the end point for any progressive social change was not far removed from radical goals for mental health care, wishing to realise a socialised and organised humanity: 'The achievement of this kindly and efficacious condition, for all patients and all societies, is the central problem of psychiatric care. It is also the central problem of social liberation.' Locating advocacy within an activism frame also intersects with consideration of power imbalances within caring relations, opening up the possibilities for alternative choices in services and the need to challenge epistemic injustices through enabling the democratic voice of service users, wherever they are to be found. It is to these activist beginnings that we now turn in the next chapter.

REFLECTIVE EXERCISES

1. Think of someone who has experienced compulsion. With reference to the different accounts discussed in this chapter – psychiatric, psychological, sociological and lay and mental health service user/survivor – identify which concepts and theories have been used (by themselves and others) to make sense of their situation.

2. In two columns make a list of the pros and cons for practising advocates having knowledge of different concepts and theories of mental health and 'illness'. Which is the most convincing and why?

3. What are the implications from these different understandings of mental health and 'illness' for how advocates approach their role and practice?

4. Consider the scope and type of care and treatment offered by contemporary mental health services in the UK. Which underlying theories of mental health and 'illness' most influence this provision?

Chapter 3

FROM MARGIN TO MAINSTREAM

A Brief Historical Overview

Introduction

This chapter critically explores the evolution of independent mental health advocacy in response to people's negative experiences of the mental health system, designed to ensure people have a voice and are able to determine what happens to them. As Chapter 5 shows, experiences of mental health services, particularly of compulsion and coercion, can disempower people and seriously compromise their confidence and ability to speak on their own behalf. Survivor activists and critical theorists have argued that the voice of people in the mental health system has been silenced on multiple grounds, including perceived irrationality (see Chapter 2). As such, independent advocacy, in its broadest sense, represents an important response to the vicissitudes of compulsion and coercion and is an adjunct to wider initiatives concerned with democratisation of services.

The definitive history of independent mental health advocacy has not yet been written, though a number of interesting sources exist (Brandon and Brandon 2000; Campbell 1996, 2005; Donnison 2009; Survivors History Group 2012). Much documentary evidence is dispersed amongst numerous groups or, indeed, lost as these have ceased to exist. Arguably, without the digitalisation and general availability of primary sources, these voices are only marginally represented in extant chronologies and histories. In this chapter, we have drawn upon these sources. Activism centred upon Manchester figures prominently in an archive preserved by Anne Plumb, who has contributed to this chapter. This is not to say that similar activities were not also occurring elsewhere, and we have endeavoured to represent the national picture and the role of key organisations. That said, some of the more local exemplars indicate the richness of relationships and alliances that are absent from much of the published material on the history of advocacy in the UK.

The chapter highlights some of the milestones in the development of what we have come to understand as mental health advocacy today. We look at key political and ideological developments and how they have shaped the notion of advocacy, the place of participation and alliances between service users and professionals.

Early origins

The language of advocacy has been traced to the fourteenth century 'Advocacie', translated as pleading for, or supporting (Jugessur and Iles 2009). This conceptualisation of the role of advocacy originated in the legal system, which has led to definitions of advocacy as 'stating a case to influence decisions, getting better services, being treated equally, being included, being protected from abuse, redressing the balance of power and becoming more aware of and exercising rights' (Jugessur and Iles 2009, p.188). These origins are clear in the development of statutory forms of advocacy including IMHA and case-based advocacy, and also go some way to accounting for the reluctance of some service users to exercise their right to an independent advocate when they already have legal representation (Ridley *et al.* 2009).

In the UK most attention has been paid to the post-war period, especially from the 1960s onward, coinciding with the rise of anti-psychiatry ideas (see Read and Wallcraft 1994). Indeed, it is difficult to contemplate any of the historical moments in the development of advocacy services without reference to the prevailing intellectual debates and policy context, which we consider in more detail in Chapter 2. Campbell (2009) also suggests that it was the confluence of policies promoting consumerism, retracting the asylum system and extant criticism of psychiatry and psychiatric services that was favourable for the growth of a survivor or service user movement, and that this, in turn, was instrumental in promoting advocacy in its various forms and, ultimately, securing rights to independent advocacy.

The legislative adoption of IMHA effectively resulted from lobbying by the Mental Health Alliance in the course of protracted debate focused on the reform of the MH Act 1983, but its path to inclusion was far from straightforward. The Expert Committee set up by the government proposed statutory advocacy framed by positive rights. The government rejected this, saying that there were sufficient voluntary advocates. Facing increasing opposition to their overall proposals, the government then used independent advocacy as a sweetener, and later threatened withdrawal before finally embedding it in the amended 2007 Act.

Some commentators argue that mental health advocacy has a long ancestry, dating back to the early seventeenth century (see Brandon and Brandon 2000; Campbell 2001). Hence, consideration of the historical roots of advocacy requires acknowledgement of the importance of contemporaneous developments across mental health services and wider society. We, therefore, identify some key points in the history of mental health advocacy but do not claim these are the final word on the history of advocacy; rather, they offer an overview or flavour of some relevant historical moments.

Recognised milestones include petitioners seeking the humane treatment of individuals, such as through the publication in 1620 of the pamphlet *The Petition of the Poor Distracted People in the House of Bedlam* or the critique of the excesses of eighteenth century Bethlem psychiatry furnished by Dr John Monroe and published in 1758. In 1816 John Haslam, alienist[1] at Bethlem, was dismissed from his post subsequent to an earlier unsuccessful court case notable for the self-advocacy of James Tilly Matthews, who disputed his diagnosed insanity. In 1845 John Perceval

---

1   Before the adoption of the role of psychiatrist, practitioners working with people in mental distress were known as alienists. This reflected a sense that individuals identified as mad were alienated from wider society and themselves.

established the Alleged Lunatics' Friend Society (ALFS), which could lay claim to being the first organisation for mental health advocacy. The ALFS was set up by a group of people after Richard Paternoster advertised in The Times for others to join him in a campaign to redress abuses in the madhouse system in 1838.

Hervey (1986) traces the roots of advocacy to 1739 when Cruden wrote an account protesting mistreatment of patients in madhouses entitled *The London Citizen Exceedingly Injured: Or a British Inquisition Displayed* (also cited by Mind 1992). More specifically, Perceval dates the foundation of the ALFS as chiefly due to Mr Luke Hansard, whose close relative was mentally disturbed. Hervey refers to the libertarian demands of the ALFS as stemming from the Magna Carta and Paineite[2] concerns with the right of individuals to certain inalienable freedoms within the welfare of society as a whole. Interestingly, liberty has re-emerged as paramount in the UN Convention on the Rights of Persons with Disabilities (Plumb 2015).

Modern milestones

The 1950s saw the commencement of policy aimed at the retraction of asylum-based mental health care and services. Implementation of so-called community care policies continued in the midst of a prominent anti-psychiatry critique during the 1960s and 1970s. Notably, radical psychiatrists in Italy led by Franco Basaglia (1964) overcame organised staff resistance and some unpopularity amongst leftist political parties in a movement to dismantle and democratise institutionalised care. Additionally, the Mental Patients Union (MPU) became active in a number of key UK locations, having been established at a meeting in 1973 as a federation of autonomous MPUs.

Similar politicised and historically situated debates and critiques were being voiced in other related contexts. The Campaign for the Mentally Handicapped (CMH) (see Ryan

---

2   Paineite refers to those influenced by the ideas of Thomas Paine, famous advocate of a politics of rights, defender of the French revolution, and influential in the American independence struggles.

with Thomas 1980) was a vocal advocacy group in the 1970s. Like Finkelstein (2007) in his Marxist analysis of disability, Ryan also believed that socio-economic changes had contributed to the segregation of people with learning difficulties. At this time, Wolfensberger's (1972a, 1972b) normalisation theory and promotion of citizen advocacy – again, largely in a learning difficulties context – was notably influential. A lesser-known publication by Wolfensberger (2005; first published 1987) constitutes a passionate polemic against the life-limiting, genocidal effects of the disempowerment of disabled people, including the impact of many standard psychiatric treatments and social antipathy towards people with mental health difficulties. This influence can be seen in the activities of, for example, North West Regional Mind when David Brandon (1981) was director, and, less obviously, in the development of the Manchester User Network that is still active. Associated with this, organisations such as The King's Fund, Good Practices in Mental Health and North West Regional Mind were all inviting service users to contribute to workshops for professionals in the early 1980s.

A particularly relevant UK application of Wolfensberger's influence can be seen in what began as the Getting to Know You Project (GTKYP) associated with Dr Judith Gray, a radical community physician, at North Manchester General Hospital. This attempt at putting normalisation principles into practice in designing innovative services (Gray 1985; Newbigging, Cadman and Westley 1989) ultimately led to the current autonomous Manchester User Network, with links to the Manchester TUC. The GTKYP led to the establishment in 1986 of a service user group at North Manchester General Hospital called 'Having a Voice', later to become the Manchester Users Support Group and, eventually, today's Manchester Users Network. Notes taken at these meetings were collated and published through the Community Psychiatric Nurses Association (1988).

The 1960s through to the 1970s was the high-water mark of the so-called anti-psychiatry movement, although perhaps it is overstating things to claim any sort of unified undertaking. This also more or less coincided with an explosion of civil rights activism and identity politics, typified in the USA in particular by Black Power, Gay Pride and Women's Liberation struggles (Tomes 2006). In many respects inspired by both anti-psychiatry and this emergent rights activism, a burgeoning patient/ex-patient/ survivor movement began to frame the excesses of psychiatry as violations of civil rights (Chamberlin 1990; McCommon 2006; Rose 1986).[3] Influential writing and thinking emerged at this time challenging the foundational constructs of psychiatry and encouraging resistance amongst survivor groupings (Spandler 2006; Thomas 2014). These works included texts readily identified as part of the constellation of explicitly anti-psychiatry thinking (even if some of the authors would have disowned such appellation) and other seminal works, notably stating feminist critiques of psychiatry and its practices (Allen 1986).

Pivotal anti-psychiatry publications included: Ronnie Laing's The Divided Self (1960) and The Politics of Experience and the Bird of Paradise (1967); Erving Goffman's Asylums (1961); Thomas Szasz's The Myth of Mental Illness (1961) and The Manufacture of Madness (1970); Michel Foucault's Madness and Civilisation (1965); Thomas Scheff's Being Mentally Ill: A Sociological Identity (1966); and Rosenhan's 'On being sane in insane places' (1973). Decisive contributions from feminist authors included: Phylis Chesler's Women and Madness (1974); various contributions in the Dorothy Smith and Sara David edited text Women Look at Psychiatry (1975); and, later, Elaine Showalter's The Female Malady: Women, Madness and English Culture, 1830–1980 (1987), Jane Ussher's Women's Madness: Misogyny or Mental Illness? (1991) and Joan Busfield's Men, Women and Madness:

---

3   The flush of liberation and related movements during the 1970s in the USA were patient/ex-patient movements. The term survivor refers not just to experiences in the psychiatric system but also to the circumstances that result in people being confined within it; Chamberlin stayed with the term ex-patient. An international organisation, Mental Health System Survivors (MHSS), however, did produce a draft policy statement which probably influenced the naming of Survivors Speak Out and the emergence in 1985 of the National Association of Psychiatric Survivors (NAPS) in the USA through individuals who were also members of MHSS.

Understanding Gender and Mental Disorder (1996). Similarly, disquiet with anomalies in the psychiatric treatment of ethnic minorities provoked further critique and attention towards alternative developments, such as transcultural psychiatry (Mercer 1986).

Contemporaneously, around the world service users and survivors were organising themselves in activist and consciousness-raising groups and producing their own writing, in their own voice. In addition to the typically identified anti-psychiatrists, the names on activists' lips were Peter R. Breggin, who later published Toxic Psychiatry (1991), and David Cohen, who later wrote, with Michael McCubbin, The Political Economy of Tardive Dyskinesia: Asymmetries in Power and Responsibility (1990), appearing in an edited collection that also included articles by Judi Chamberlin and Leonard Frank, long-time campaigner against electroshock treatment.

More often than not, survivor activism was identified with, and proselytised for, different forms of advocacy (Chamberlin 1990). Influential centres of activity in the USA and Canada, for example, produced dynamic and creative magazines and pamphlets such as *Phoenix Rising* in Toronto.[4] This survivor activism was pioneered by the likes of Judi Chamberlin in Boston, affiliated to the Mental Patients Liberation Front, and culminating in the breakthrough text *On Our Own: Patient-Controlled Alternatives to the Mental Health System* (Chamberlin 1978). Chamberlin coined the term 'mentalism' to denote discriminatory practices against psychiatrised persons. The more progressive elements within anti-psychiatry discourse chimed with a notable left-leaning or Marxist disposition amongst many early survivor groupings (Thomas 2014). The history of these times and subsequent movement activism is well told in Linda Morrison's (2005) book *Talking Back to Psychiatry*.

Despite the marked influence on movement politics and to some extent amongst professional mental health academics and practitioners (most training courses at the very least offer a nod

---

4   Now digitised and archived at www.psychiatricsurvivorarchives.com/ phoenix.html by the Psychiatric Survivor Archives of Toronto.

to anti-psychiatry texts), anti-psychiatry ideas were also open to criticism. For many commentators, the degree of enablement afforded to survivor movement activism has been overstated in some quarters, with little actual impact upon psychiatric practices (Campbell 1989). With hindsight, perhaps the most significant and lasting contribution was to open up the space for critical debate around the value of psychiatry and the nature of psychiatric services.

Peter Sedgwick's (1982) later, equally powerful contribution *Psychopolitics* debunked many of the key players of the anti-psychiatry critique for poor scholarly practices and neglect of more broadly cast political analyses. Sedgwick operated at the intersection of survivor and left-wing labour movement activism, and as such was interested in the alienating features of psychiatry for all concerned – patients and staff – and the potential for better informed alliances between worker and survivor interest groups. Indeed, the history of the service user and survivor movement in the UK is replete with examples of such alliances and constructive cooperation between professionals sympathetic to movement goals and service user and survivor activists (Beeforth *et al.* 1990; Campbell and Lindow 1997; Thomas 2014). Some of these ideas have been taken up recently as of continued relevance to both survivor and trade union organising in contemporary times (Cresswell and Spandler 2009; McKeown *et al.* 2014b). Without claiming significant impact upon workplace culture, the trade union UNISON and Mind collaborated on the production of *Guidelines on Advocacy for Mental Health Workers*, written by survivor activists Jim Read and Jan Wallcraft (1994), also producing booklets directed at NHS union members focused on empowerment and equalities.

Whilst the 1980s saw the rise of New Right social policy, ushering in health service reforms and cutbacks in funding, various groups such as the British Network for Alternatives to Psychiatry (BNAP) and Campaign Against Psychiatric Oppression (CAPO) became active.

The 1988 Griffiths Report, for example, which heralded the policy of community care, was replete with the individualism of the time, proposing: 'giving people a greater individual say in how they live their lives and the services they need to help them do so'. This led to the NHS and Community Care Act 1990 which first introduced the idea of an internal market into the NHS, but also included intentions for public consultation and service user involvement in planning and delivery of care. Critics bemoaned the limited version of involvement on offer, which arguably maintained service users in a largely passive role, delivering a watered-down version of the proposals in the preceding White Paper (Walker 1989). Despite this, Barnes and Cotterell (2012) saw this policy turn as influential in various attempts to meaningfully encourage service users' voice, described in Goss and Miller's (1995) *From Margin to Mainstream*. Out of the involvement of survivors/service users with authorities in the 1980s, service user critiques arose (e.g. Lindow 1991), exposing difficulties with, and guidelines for, 'partnership' and 'service user involvement'. This, despite personal and practical issues for service user representatives and inherent structural problems (Campbell 1996).

In this period, there were a number of damning reports and inquiries into service failings in mental health, notably in secure settings, culminating in the 1992 *Public Inquiry into Complaints About Ashworth Special Hospital* chaired by Louis Blom Cooper. Exposing serious abuses of patients, this recommended the establishment of an independent advocacy service. The Ashworth CAB Patients Advocacy Service (ACPAS) was set up in 1993 and was the first formal service of its kind in a high security hospital in the UK (Bamber 2007).[5] Prior to this date, and influential in the course of the first Ashworth Inquiry, was the establishment of an office of WISH (Women in Special Hospitals, later to become Women in Secure Hospitals) on the hospital site, and

---

5   The Manchester MPU, in the 1980s, were involved with what was then Moss Side High Security Hospital (eventually incorporated into Ashworth Hospital). They also had an office in Prestwich Hospital (medium secure); the contact was a nurse – Manchester MPU was not limited to patients/ex-patients.

organising collective advocacy for detained women (McCabe 1996; Stevenson 1989).

The desirability of service user involvement, empowerment and participation, at least at the level of rhetoric, continued to be expressed in multiple waves of health and mental health policy, continuing to the present day. Arguably, this distinctly consumerist policy context was helpful for autonomous self-advocacy activity, which also grew in these otherwise not so auspicious times. It is paradoxical that the Conservative Government's Task Force on Mental Health responded to demands from Survivors Speak Out, MindLink and UK Advocacy Network reps and provided funds for 16 regional service user conferences and publications which included a code of practice for advocacy (Conlan and Day 1994).[6] Indeed, Pilgrim and Ramon (2009) note the marked continuities in policy despite electoral changes from Conservative to New Labour, these being understandable in terms of a neo-liberal hegemony, with individualism squeezing out contemplation of social models of mental distress and collective approaches to advocacy.

Survivor activism and advocacy

Certain key local and national developments can be seen to have played a significant role in the establishment of IMHA in the UK, and illustrate the complex dynamics between survivor activism, patient councils, collective advocacy and more individualised, independent forms.

The Survivors History website provides detail regarding milestones and influences on the intertwined growth of survivor activism and mental health advocacy. This archive of user-led publications and other materials notes the 1981 genesis of the Advocacy Alliance set up by the Spastics Society, Mencap, Mind, One to One and the Leonard Cheshire Foundation following the broadcast of *Silent Minority*, a shocking documentary showing institutional abuses of vulnerable individuals. This collective

---

6   Others focused on a charter for users of mental health services, and training service users as trainers, speakers and workshop facilitators.

aspired to 'give the most vulnerable and forgotten patients in mentally handicapped hospitals a friend and an advocate', and 'provide long-term friendship, emotional support and advice for patients. It will uphold their human rights and statutory entitlements, prevent abuse and neglect and ensure access to a high quality of educational, housing, health and social services'.[7] A persuasive case can be made that the roots of contemporary notions of independent advocacy were in user movement politicking associated with groups like the Nottingham Advocacy Group (NAG), Survivors Speak Out (SSO) and other local forums and initiatives across the country. Peter Campbell (2009) recalls the autumn of 1985 as a time when

> the concept of self-advocacy was emerging...the invention of professionals, or at least the professional journals. In the space of eighteen months or so, it had taken over to such an extent that people in user groups – people like myself – began to accept that what we were doing was indeed 'self-advocacy'. (p.206)

Over the years, without there ever necessarily being a single, unified UK service user/survivor movement, there have been moments of distinct activism for the establishment of advocacy independent of psychiatric services, and advocacy in its campaigning form has always been a characteristic of survivor movement politics (Barker and Peck 1987). Perhaps most notable in this lineage of activism is the history of NAG, emerging in the mid-1980s and appreciatively described in a couple of detailed accounts (Barnes 2007; Barnes and Gell 2012). Seeded by exposure to proselytisers of European models of patient councils at a key international mental health conference in Brighton in 1985, a grouping of service user activists, affiliated academics, Mind volunteers and law centre personnel convened the Nottingham Patients' Council Support Group (NPCSG), which was later to turn into NAG.

This conference developed the Mental Health Charter 2000 Action programmes for a World in Crisis – the Brighton

---

7   Cited on the Survivors History website at http://studymore.org.uk/ mhhglo.htm#advocacyUK (accessed on 6 April 2015).

Declaration on the Rights of Mentally Ill People and the Promotion of Mental Health. A group of activists also set up their own Declaration Group on Self and Citizen Advocacy and wrote the section on Self-determination as a Human Right: Its Implication for 'Mental Health Services'. This was a clear example of collective advocacy, and there is arguably still a long way to go to meet these demands made in 1985. Little attention has been paid to charters that were collectively decided, and as to local social services' mission statements, one activist commented at the time that he was collecting and exchanging these like football stickers! These user-defined charters scarcely entered into the realm of professionals and, as mentioned earlier, may have now been pushed aside by policies framed around individualism.

In Nottingham, patient councils were set up in both the County and City hospitals, but relations with staff and psychiatrists were turbulent, and NPCSG were soon banned from the County hospital. Barnes and Gell (2012) marvellously evoke the mood of solidarity amongst patients at the time, depicting the attendance at the first patient council meeting in the City hospital as akin to 'workers downing tools in a factory and marching to trades union meetings' (p.19).

The early NAG was an amalgam of support for patient councils, issue-based individual advocacy and more longer-term citizen advocacy. Barnes and Gell remark upon the clear links with national groups such as SSO,[8] opening up campaigning and protest endeavours, and the renaming of Mind's National Consumer Advisory Network as MindLink in 1991, providing for user voice within Mind. Thomas (2014) notes the Channel 4 broadcast of *We're Not Mad We're Angry* in 1986, featuring prominent SSO activists such as Peter Campbell and Jan Wallcraft

---

8   Survivors Speak Out distributed Crisis Cards naming an advocate and details on Advance Directives on the initiative of a prominent member of SSO, Mike Lawson, who with his partner set up an International Self Advocacy Alliance in 1989. These cards were reissued by the Lambeth Link Advocacy Project, which also developed an extended version, Charter '90, of the Hackney Mental Health Action Group's Charter on the Rights of People with Mental Distress (1986).

and with a high degree of editorial control, as a key milestone for critical ideas reaching a wider audience.

NAG also organised the conference which led to the formation of the United Kingdom Advocacy Network (UKAN) to support a national growth in local advocacy groups, with NAG and UKAN touring the country promoting advocacy. Crossley (2006) comments on the pivotal role of UKAN in this regard, and how the features of their networking and support activity in the promotion of advocacy were resonant with characteristics of movement politics and organising. He makes particular reference to the use of packs and structural support in conjunction with SSO, complemented with mailshots and newsletters, all of which helped a growing advocacy community to thrive and inter-connect, sharing ideas for practice and development.

NAG explicitly appreciated a link between collective and individual advocacy by framing service users as active citizens, rather than simply consumers of health care services (Barnes and Gell 2012). Towards the end of this period of advocacy expansion Marius Romme and Sandra Escher published *Accepting Voices* (1993) and engaged in various meetings and conferences promoting the ideas which culminated in establishment of the Hearing Voices Network (HVN). The significant event for activists was the meeting in 1987 for voice hearers organised by Romme, his patient and the presenter of a radio programme. In 1988 a national meeting was organised jointly by Foundation Response, a self-help organisation of people who hear voices, and the Limburg Department of Social Psychiatry, to which professionals were invited. Conferences have continued ever since, leading to the international organisation Intervoice.

For the duration of NAG's existence there was dissatisfaction amongst workers and volunteers with the level of interest sustained on the part of NHS personnel and organisations in advocacy, patient councils or even consistently attending meetings. There was also some internal turbulence, sometimes turning on differences over conceptions of advocacy but exacerbated along the way by funding shortfalls and cuts. After two decades of consistent advocacy provision, periods of expansion and diversification, and engagement in nationwide evangelism for user/survivor movement politics and the value of advocacy, NAG lost the contracts to deliver advocacy across Nottingham and was defunct by 2010 (Barnes and Gell 2012).

Notable later developments include the establishment in 2001 of Advocacy Across London, which later became the national Action for Advocacy (A4A) organisation in 2003. This influential grouping supported networking and knowledge sharing amongst advocacy services and advocates and played an important leadership role in key debates, not least on the professionalising agenda for advocacy, including interest in training and quality standards (Action for Advocacy 2006). These organisations also published the unique advocacy magazine *Planet Advocacy*.

The mental health charity Mind has maintained a longstanding interest in advocacy, publishing a pocket guide as early as 1992, advocacy standards in 2006 and a practical guide in 2000, revised in 2010 and available online. The 1992 Guide is an interesting historical document that tells some of the history of different forms of advocacy, including the crucial link to activism through groups such as MPU, SSO and NAG. This text neatly makes clear the value of independent advocacy, stressing the conflict of loyalties and interests for professional staff such as nurses. Also noted is the pioneering work since the 1970s by Mind's London Legal Department, offering some degree of specialised representation and advice. The Guide points out that, as far back as 1983, European law on minimum standards for civil detention was framed such that the principle of independent advocacy provision should be adhered to, but the UK government failed to agree. William Bingley, in his post as Legal Director of Mind, and Larry Gostin[9] (1990) before him,

---

9 Gostin also provided an influential critique in the course of the replacement of the MH Act 1959 with the MH Act 1983, and proposed that there should be patient advocates located in hospitals to limit professional responsibility and protect patients against 'the tendency to impose their views on unwilling patients' based on the experience of a system in New Jersey where a large number of lawyers were employed to act in this capacity (Bluglass 1984, p.130).

were instrumental in shaping Mind's interest in advocacy[10] and aligning it with campaigning pressure on government for more humane services and administration of legislation (McKeown 2012a, 2012b). Bingley also co-authored the 1983 Mental Health Act Code of Practice and was instrumental in setting up the first undergraduate course for mental health advocates at the University of Central Lancashire in 2000.

Advocacy as a right

The eventual implementation of IMHA services can be seen to have resulted directly from campaigning and organising in relation to the reform process for the Mental Health Act. Prominent in this was the Mental Health Alliance, formed in 1999 as a coalition of movement groups, major mental health voluntary sector organisations and mental health staff and professional associations and unions[11] and a long-running consultation process initiated by the government's convening of the expert panel chaired by Genevra Richardson. Playing into these deliberations were wider concerns about the quality of mental health services, issues of public protection and risk (amplified by a number of high-profile service failures, such as the homicide of Jonathan Zito), and acknowledgement that opportunities for advocacy, self-advocacy and service user involvement were unevenly distributed.

A review of local UK service user groups highlighted some problems with diversity, most such groups' membership failing to proportionately include people from ethnic minorities (Wallcraft, Read and Sweeney 2003). Though efforts have been

---

10 Campaigning US lawyers, such as Michael Perlin, were also influential in framing mental health rights in a wider libertarian, civil rights context.

11 Towards the end of the reform process these staff organisations split from the alliance, forming their own grouping to more assertively represent professional interests, largely precipitated by concerns over the Approved Mental Health Practitioner (AMHP) role (AMICUS et al. 2007).

made to establish a BAME service user/survivor movement, this has been starved of funding and recognition (Thomas 2014). Amongst BAME communities, with growing dissatisfaction with mainstream psychiatric services and recognition that Black men in particular were over-represented in in-patient care and increasingly detained within secure units, a number of alternative mental health services were established[12] (Francis *et al.* 1989). These often also organised advocacy services. Notable examples are Sharing Voices, Bradford; Equalities National Council, London; African Caribbean Mental Health Services, Manchester; and Mary Seacole House and The Advocacy Project in Liverpool. Such advocacy was often sceptical of the emphasis placed upon models of independence, preferring to reflect cultures of inter-dependence.

Impact of political ideology

Arguably, the more radical politics of an energised user movement was able to capitalise upon the space opened up by the espousal of consumerism contained within New Right politics, which have persisted in some form or other since the election of Margaret Thatcher in 1979. With Thatcherism came an acceleration of the Mental Hospital retraction process, and the previously mentioned policy embrace of Care in the Community. Critics suggest that this was as much motivated by cost as it was by concerns for the welfare of the institutionalised (Means, Richards and Smith 2008). Corollary activity saw a general retreat from the ideology of State provision of welfare: the diminution of the so-called 'Nanny State'.

Somewhat paradoxically, these consumerist measures were not antithetical to service user activism, and could be seen to foreground notions of patient choice and involvement rhetoric. The downsizing of various sectors of the welfare state led to a growth in independent sector provision, with a significant

---

12   Paradoxically a grievance at an SSO AGM held in Birmingham was that the Black community was being denied access to the wider mental health services available to the White population.

proportion of this being amongst voluntary agencies. The prevailing political ethos was framed around individual freedom of choice and consumerism in all domains, including health. Notwithstanding criticism that the architects of this ideological shift were erroneously applying free-market principles in an inappropriate context, and that 'more choice' actually translated into 'less choice', there had been undoubted problems in the NHS. For example, the evidence of the Black Report (Department of Health and Social Security 1980) into health inequalities seriously challenged the extent to which socialised medicine had tackled issues of equity.

Similarly, regardless of one's ideological persuasion, the NHS at the time could be criticised for a lack of responsiveness to diverse needs. To this extent, expansion in the voluntary sector suggested the potential to improve sensitivity to target groups with special needs. There was also a problem in terms of resource allocation with a well-documented 'inverse-care law' where the most needy were less likely to access services (Tudor Hart 1971). The promotion of consumer choice and rights would arguably address some of these issues.

The government rhetoric of New Labour urged concerted efforts to ensure service user and carer voices were heard at all levels of relevant organisations. The associated debate replaced a simple notion of consumerism with the concept of participation privileged as the route to empowerment of service users. For Barnes and Bowl (2001, p.166):

> Whatever the limitations of the official rhetoric of partnership, this is a more useful starting point for the development of empowerment strategies than that offered by an appeal to consumer choice. Partnership has the capacity to offer something of value to both user and provider of services by placing greater responsibilities on both to engage in a new type of relationship.

In parallel with these developments, an emerging rhetorical shift in clinical mental health practice towards an acceptance of notions of therapeutic alliances perhaps provides a more promising context for the positive development of advocacy. Such alliances are relationships based upon participatory processes of shared decision making. Crucial to this approach is the extent to which individuals feel empowered to engage with the process, such that their authentic voice is heard in the dialogue that constructs care. Latterly, such initiatives have clustered around organising principles of recovery, and have been badged as co-production.

Despite the progressive tenor of various associated policy pronouncements, and some undoubted progress on the ground, many service users remain sceptical that the actual quality of service provision matches the policy rhetoric, this sense being compounded by increasing levels of compulsion and coercion. Other commentators understand this in terms of contradictory policy aims of humane care and social control, reserving particular criticism for in-patient units (Pilgrim and Ramon 2009). Factoring in the perception amongst many advocates and advocacy organisations that relationships with staff and care teams can often leave a lot to be desired, then much work remains to be done to truly embed high-quality independent advocacy into the routine delivery of mental health care (see Chapter 11 for more on staff relationships with advocacy).

Conclusions

The link between the historical development of advocacy and user movement politics in some way reflects Campbell's (2009) view of a journey from 'margin to mainstream'. This movement activism contribution is inextricably linked to the critique of psychiatry presented in Chapter 2. Moreover, the achievement of a legally supported right to independent advocacy was an undoubted achievement of the service user/survivor movement, and arguably could not have been realised without this activism.

REFLECTIVE EXERCISES

1. Make a list of the main historical strands in the development of independent mental health advocacy. Highlight any that you consider to be of key significance. How do these impact on independent mental health advocacy today?

2. Map independent mental health advocacy provision in your locality. Research the link between service user/survivor activity (past or current) and local independent advocacy provision. How strong or weak are these links? What can you learn from this?

3. Appreciating the past history and development of independent mental health advocacy, what lessons can be learnt that may inform future developments?

4. Keeping in mind the main historical strands discussed in the chapter, perform a SWOT (strengths, weaknesses, opportunities and threats) analysis of independent mental health advocacy provision. What does this tell you about its future prospects?

Chapter 4

MENTAL HEALTH ADVOCACY, RIGHTS AND THE LAW

Introduction

Legislation and policy provide an essential safeguard to ensure that human rights are upheld for all citizens so that everyone can reach the goals of 'full citizenship, equality and human dignity' as demanded by service user movements (Chamberlin 1998, p.408). The extent to which this is compromised by the existence of a legal framework for involuntary admission and treatment is widely debated, as sectioning strips people of aspects of their personal autonomy (Barnes, Bowl and Fisher 1990). As referred to in the previous chapter, this debate was very evident in the process of reforming the MH Act 1983, which took place in England and Wales over a ten-year period from 1997. Any consideration of the roots of IMHA needs to be cognisant of the birth pangs of the MH Act 2007, so this chapter provides a critical reflection on mental health law to illuminate potential ambiguities and conflicts inherent in the IMHA role. We start by considering the emergence of statutory advocacy in England via the amended MH Act 2007, pausing to reflect on the standard ethical justification for detention and compulsory treatment. We consider controversies surrounding the review of the MH Act 1983 and the origins of IMHA as the product of that debate, emerging as a statutory mechanism for protecting rights. A summary of the role of IMHAs and the duties on public services to make them available is discussed before we explore the framing of IMHA within a discourse of rights, distinguishing between positive and negative rights. We argue that the introduction of IMHA reflects the narrow conception of human rights within the MH Act 2007, acknowledging that the application of human rights to the mental health context has been somewhat problematic. We conclude by arguing that IMHAs have an important role to play in pursuing positive rights, wider than the legal obligations, and this may place them in a difficult position vis à vis mental health services that are narrowly focused and underpinned by limited considerations of 'best interests'.

Advocacy and the law

In a global context, advocacy is identified as a fundamental element of the mental health system (WHO 2003), although this typically refers to collective advocacy or advocacy on behalf of people with mental health problems to promote their cause. The incorporation of advocacy on behalf of individuals into law and policy has developed hand in hand in England with a policy impetus to develop care and support that is person centred. This increased focus on individuals and drive towards consumerism is critiqued as reflecting a neo-liberal agenda ideology in the previous chapter.

However, there are two issues that cannot be ignored and to which advocacy can offer a potential partial remedy. First, the relative powerlessness of people in their encounter with services. The vulnerability of individuals within health and social care services is a recurrent theme and has again been highlighted by the recent publication of several reports pointing to neglect, abuse and avoidable deaths as a consequence of the behaviour of staff and indifference of services to the views and voices of service users and their families (Department of Health 2012; Francis 2013). Second, inequities in the access to and use of health and social care services favour people with greater resources (money, education, social capital), compounding the social disadvantage of some groups. The potential of advocacy has, therefore, been promoted by successive governments – for example, by Phil

Hope, the Minister for State for Social Care in 2009 – in a mental health context:

> Advocacy is one way of helping to ensure that the patient and patients' needs are at the heart of the health service and to drive forward quality of care. Giving patients a voice through advocacy or in other ways is about more than simply improving services, although it will have that effect... Advocacy is about helping preserve a person's dignity and self-respect, as well as protecting their legal and human rights. (Hansard 2009, column 109)

Advocacy framed as a form of protection and a mechanism to ensure that people's views are heard in decision making about their care has, thus, been incorporated into English law. Statutory advocacy, as illustrated in Table 4.1, had its genesis in representation of complaints, was extended through the MC Act to decision making, the brief widened by the introduction of IMHA and most through the Care Act 2014 to strengthen involvement in care planning processes for adult social care. As discussed in the previous chapter, other types of advocacy exist, and this poses questions about the nature of statutory advocacy, its purpose, and how different forms of advocacy relate to each other.

TABLE 4.1 THE LEGAL FRAMEWORK FOR STATUTORY ADVOCACY

Date	Legal instrument	Type of advocacy	Definition of advocacy and its function
2002	Adoption and Children Act	Representation of complaints under the 1989 Children Act	To support care leavers and children making a complaint under the 1989 Children Act.
2003	Health and Social Care (Community Health and Standards) Act	Independent Complaints Advocacy Service (ICAS)	To enable people to make a complaint about the National Health Service.
2005	Mental Capacity Act (MC Act)	Independent Mental Capacity Advocates (IMCAs)	To support people (aged 16 and over) who lack capacity to make certain decisions, relating to either • serious medical treatment or • long-term moves (more than 28 days in hospital/8 weeks in care home).

cont.

Date	Legal instrument	Type of advocacy	Definition of advocacy and its function
2007	Mental Health (Amendment) Act 2007	Independent Mental Health Advocates (IMHAs)	To protect the rights of people detained under the MH Act 1983 and provide an additional safeguard by helping qualifying patients to obtain and understand information about the legal provisions to which they are subject, the rights and safeguards to which they are entitled, and help those patients exercise their rights through supporting participation in decision making.
2007	Deprivation of Liberty Safeguards (DOLS)	Relevant persons representative service for people subject to DOLS authorisations[1]	To maintain contact with the relevant person and: • represent and support the relevant person in all matters relating to DOLS, including, if appropriate, requesting a review, using an organisation's complaints procedure on the person's behalf or making an application to the Court of Protection • to provide support that is independent of the relevant person's commissioners and service providers.
2014	Care Act	Independent advocacy	To facilitate the involvement of people who either have • substantial difficulty in being involved in assessments, care and support planning, and reviews or • where there is no one available to act on the person's behalf.

1 This could be provided by advocacy services but is a distrinct role. See SCIE (2015) for further information.

In the context of statutory advocacy, there has been confusion concerning the relationship between the MH Act 1983, MC Act 2005 and DOLS, which the revised Code of Practice seeks to clarify (Department of Health 2015). Both the MH Act 1983 and the MC Act 2005 apply to the care and treatment of adults who lack capacity and both were amended by the MH Act 2007, which added provisions relating to DOLS, first introduced as part of the MC Act 2005. The legislation allows people to be deprived of their liberty, where following an independent assessment it is judged to be necessary in their best interests, and DOLS are the measures that apply in such instances. People can be detained under the MH Act, whether or not they have capacity to consent, and in general the MH Act 'trumps' the MC Act (Herlihy and Holloway 2009, p.479) and must be used if the person has made a valid and applicable advance decision refusing treatment. In the context of the MC Act 2005, capacity is assumed unless proven otherwise and the provisions of the Act relate to treatment for medical conditions, other than mental health, and to decisions relating to place of residence. It has been argued that separate mental health legislation is intrinsically discriminatory and that mental capacity legislation with additional safeguards should be sufficient for non-consensual treatment of both mental and physical health conditions (Szmukler, Daw and Dawson 2010; Zigmond 1998). However, mental health professionals successfully rebutted this on the basis that the criteria to define capacity are narrowly focused on cognitive ability, arguing that people whose decision-making capacity is significantly impaired as a result of mental disorder should not be excluded from non-consensual treatment (Zigmond 2008). Consequently, IMHAs have a role in relation to people who are subject to compulsion under the MH Act who have capacity, but may not consent to proposed treatment, *and* people who lack capacity, with advocacy in such instances termed 'non-instructed advocacy'.

Mental health law in England and Wales

In most countries, the state has powers to detain people with mental health problems and, in specific circumstances, treat them against their will. Existing mental health legislation brings together two strands of law that originated in the eighteenth century (Moncrieff 2003b). The first is the power of the state to detain people judged to be 'dangerous' enacted in the Vagrancy Acts of 1713 and 1744 (Bluglass 1984; Moncrieff 2003b). The second is the concern of the state to protect patients' interests, with the Regulation of Private Madhouses Act of 1774 providing for the regulation of private asylums and introducing the requirement of certification by a doctor for detention (Moncrieff 2003b; Porter 1990).

Overview of the Mental Health Act 2007

The current legal framework for detention and compulsion in England is the MH Act 1983, amended by the MH Act 2007.

One of the major amendments relates to the definition of mental disorder. The previous definition outlined four forms of mental disorder (mental illness, mental impairment, severe mental impairment and psychopathic disorder) was replaced with 'any disorder or disability of the mind'. Although this was couched as a simplification, it has been criticised for widening the definition of mental disorder and, therefore, broadening the scope of the MH Act.

There are four forms of compulsion under the Act: detention, supervised community treatment, conditional discharge and guardianship. Detention is the most common form of compulsion and there are two main types: detention under Section 2, which allows a person to be detained in hospital for assessment for up to 28 days, and under Section 3, allowing for detention in hospital for treatment, for up to six months initially, which can then be renewed for another six months and then after that for up to a year at a time.[2] Detention means that a person is unable to leave

---

2   Various other sections relate to detention in secure units subsequent to involvement in the criminal justice system.

the hospital without permission, and the criteria for detention under Sections 2 and 3 are summarised in Box 4.1.

BOX 4.1 CRITERIA FOR DETENTION UNDER SECTIONS 2 AND 3
Criteria for detention under Section 2

The criteria are:

- the person is suffering from a mental disorder of a nature or degree that warrants assessment in hospital for assessment (or assessment followed by treatment) for at least a limited period

- they ought to be detained in the interest of their health and safety, or the protection of others.

Criteria for detention under Section 3

The criteria are:

- the person is suffering from a mental disorder of a nature or degree which makes it appropriate for them to receive treatment in hospital

- it is necessary for their health and safety, or for the protection of others, that they should receive treatment

- treatment cannot be provided unless they are detained under Section 3

- appropriate medical treatment is available for them.

(Source: Department of Health 2015, p.113)

Imposing restrictions on people's liberty is obviously a highly serious matter: it has civil liberties implications and potentially infringes human rights. As the following chapter illustrates, it has a profound emotional and social impact, undermining self-worth, leading to feelings of violation (Katsakou and Priebe 2007) and damaging a sense of identity and personal integrity (Gault 2009; Johansson and Lundman 2002). 'It also challenges the foundation of modern-day clinical practice – that of informed consent' (Fistein *et al.* 2009, p.47). Therefore, legal frameworks for detention and compulsion aim to provide safeguards to protect patients' rights. In the case of mental health law in England and Wales, this includes rights to information, to refuse specific treatments, which may not apply in certain circumstances, access to Mental Health Tribunals (MHTs), which have the power to discharge if the criteria for detention are not met, and rights to access an IMHA. Furthermore, monitoring of the use of the Act is mandated to the Care Quality Commission.[3] We now consider the complexity of the ethical and legal context in which IMHAs are operating.

Ethical justifications for detention and compulsion

Mental health legislation is the focus for activism internationally, with the involuntary detention and treatment of people experiencing mental health problems seen as a fundamental breach of human rights. The standard ethical justification for detention and compulsion hinges on consideration of the principle of respect for autonomy, one of four ethical principles claimed to underpin all health care:

> To respect an autonomous agent is, first, to recognize that person's capacities and perspectives, including his or her right to hold views and to make choices, and to take actions based on personal values and beliefs. The moral demand that we respect the autonomy of persons can be expressed as a principle of respect for autonomy, which should be stated as involving both a negative obligation and a positive obligation. As a negative obligation autonomous actions should not be subject to the controlling constraints by others. As a positive

---

3   This function was undertaken by the Mental Health Act Commission until 2009.

obligation, this principle requires both respectful treatment in disclosing information and actions that foster autonomous decision-making. (Beauchamp 2007, p.4)

From this standpoint, mental illness is seen as limiting personal autonomy and capacity for decision making as an autonomous agent, and therefore legislating for involuntary detention and treatment becomes justified as a means of restoring autonomy. The case for involuntary detention and treatment is typically made on the basis that the person's interests and autonomy in the longer term are protected by overriding their autonomy in the short term (Schopp 1993). For this to be meaningful, however, the principle of reciprocity is evoked such that, if people's civil liberties are to be curtailed, this must be matched by rights to treatment and adequate quality of resources (Eastman 1994). Equally, it implies that the means of restricting individual autonomy must be the least restrictive possible. In potential tension with the principle of respect for autonomy is the principle of beneficence, which relates to helping others by preventing or removing possible harms, often referred to as paternalism, providing the rationale underpinning 'best interest judgments'. This involves balancing benefits and risks, not only to the individual but wider society (Beauchamp 2007), as reflected in the criteria for Sections 2 and 3, described earlier.

The tension between these two principles – respect for autonomy and beneficence – are at the heart of many ethical debates within health care. It raises the question, in the mental health care context, of whether people should be treated involuntarily to alleviate their distress and, if justified, whether this ought to apply equally to people with physical health problems (Saks 2003). Consequently, in relation to people with mental health problems, the ethical arguments for detention and compulsion primarily focus on two tenets: first, the competence, often termed capacity, of the individual to make decisions and, second, the risk to self or others from the individual, with the latter shaping much of the discourse.

If competence becomes a criterion, then people with mental health problems are treated no differently than people with physical health problems, whose autonomy is overridden when they are not competent, for example the lifesaving treatment of an unconscious person (Saks 2003). However, such an argument ignores psychiatry's preoccupation with rationality and the individual self (Bracken and Thomas 2001) and mental illness-related stigma. Arguably, psychiatric demarcations of irrationality constitute forms of epistemic violence, with people with mental health problems excluded from spheres of legitimate knowledge (Liegghio 2013). In other words, people with mental health problems, particularly at times of acute distress, are likely to be judged incompetent because the dominant frame of reference privileges a particular view of rationality and biomedical explanations for their distress.

The second tenet relating to the risk of harm to self and others is also the focus of controversy and, although not seen on its own as sufficient grounds for compulsion and detention in law, has exercised a profound influence on both mental health law, policy and practice in England for the past 150 years (Pilgrim 2007).[4] Psychiatric and lay depictions of irrationality contribute to an 'othering' of those deemed to be mentally disordered, a process which feeds into public fears of dangerous madness and also, arguably, the framing of mental health legislation by governments with an ambivalent concern for an anxious electorate (McKeown and Stowell-Smith 2006).

Such issues formed a focus for dispute during the reform of the MH Act 1983 and provide the basis for conflict between IMHAs and mental health professionals: self-determination or best interests? We explore this further in Chapter 11.

Reform of the Mental Health Act 1983

In 1993, proposals were discussed for the reform of the MH Act 1983 with a call for radical reform involving a principled approach to formulating new legislation rather than the 'considered

---

4   Whether preventive detention without the presence of mental disorder could ever be used has been debated (see Campbell and Heginbotham 1991).

pragmatism' of the 1959 and 1983 Acts (Eastman 1994, p.43). Such principles would include those of: reciprocity; promotion of self-determination; services designed for individuals; least restriction; close proximity of services; protection from neglect, exploitation and abuse; and people subject to compulsion taking all the decisions of which they are capable (Eastman 1994, p.43). It was to be another five years before the English government formally announced its intention to reform the MH Act 1983, shortly after New Labour came to power, with the publication of the Green Paper *Modernising Mental Health Services: Safe, Sound and Supportive* (Department of Health 1998). Alongside a discourse of the inadequacy of community care, the focus clearly shifted during the 1990s from concerns about the welfare of people with mental health problems in long-stay institutions to concerns about risk and the threat posed to public safety by people with a mental illness (Goodwin 1997). Although notions of risk management were evident in the MH Act 1983, in its restriction of detention on the grounds of safety to self or others (Maden 2007), ensuring public safety from dangerous individuals was a major driver for New Labour's policy direction, reflecting a sentiment amongst Ministers that non-compliance was no longer an option (Zigmond 2001).

Subsequent to the announcement of the government's intentions to reform the MH Act, there followed a report from an Expert Committee, chaired by Professor Genevra Richardson, charged with making recommendations. Notably, the key principles underlying the group's proposals were those of non-discrimination and patient autonomy along with the importance of user participation and consensual care. Furthermore, the principle of reciprocity was promoted such that health and social care authorities should be placed under a duty to provide an appropriate standard of care and treatment for those subject to compulsion (Department of Health 1999). The Committee also proposed the right to advocacy, at the earliest possible opportunity, and the right to information about and assistance with drawing up an advance directive. Many of the Richardson Committee proposals were rejected by the government in the subsequent Green Paper. Unsurprisingly, this draft Bill, published in 2002, met with a hostile reception from user groups and many professionals, including senior psychiatrists, represented in the membership of the Mental Health Alliance who were united in their opposition to the proposals, seen as legislating for compulsion for the few rather than care for the many[5] (Pilgrim 2007). In particular, concerns were expressed about the breadth of criteria for non-consensual treatment, the approach to people with a diagnosis of 'dangerous, severe personality disorder' and the extension of compulsory powers to people living in the community[6] (Wright 2002). Arguments were made for the new legislation to focus on positive rights, early intervention and access to appropriate services and support to prevent the need for compulsory powers. Concern for the liberties and rights of individuals caught up in the mental health system and affinity for the existence of effectively resourced and independent advocacy was a key part of this discourse. For the first time, a statutory right to advocacy was included in the White Paper and this was warmly welcomed (Wright 2002), with the Department of Health commissioning a study to identify what this specialist advocacy should look like (Barnes, Brandon and Webb 2002).

As a consequence of the opposition to the draft Bill, the government undertook a series of roadshows to consult with stakeholders and a revised draft Bill was published in 2004. This also met with disapproval (Mental Health Alliance 2005), and was criticised as 'fundamentally flawed' following scrutiny by a Joint Committee of Parliament (Joint Committee on the Draft Mental Health Bill 2005). In respect of advocacy, the Joint Committee commented that 'the overwhelming weight of evidence received

---

5   Letter to *The Guardian*, 19 November 1999, p.25.

6   Interestingly, Tory politician Virginia Bottomley eventually backtracked on Community Supervision/Treatment Orders (first proposed by the British Association of Social Workers, believing that it would be better for people to be treated in the community rather than in hospital), while New Labour reinstated them despite Tessa Jowell, in 1993, stating that the Secretary of State should not be 'panicked into taking measures in order to appease what may be a tide of public apprehension' (*The Guardian*, 8 July 1993).

endorsed the provision of an advocacy service' (p.121). Their response, however, was critical of the government's proposals and pointed to the importance of adequate funding to translate the right to access advocacy into reality, otherwise it would remain a meaningless ambition. They, therefore, recommended that local authorities and health authorities be placed under a statutory duty to produce local plans for the development and funding of independent health advocacy services to meet the needs of all service users, including mental health service users. Furthermore, the Joint Committee recognised the importance of the proposed advocacy services complementing, and not disrupting, existing advocacy services, and provision to a wider group of mental health service users than detained patients. They recommended access to advocacy at the earliest possible opportunity, for example as soon as detention is proposed, and ensuring that children under the age of 16 had the same safeguards as adults, including advocacy.

The government published its response to the Joint Committee's scrutiny of their proposals and disagreed with many. Of particular note was the rejection of the Committee's recommendations that the legislation should be about improving service provision, framing it as a legal process for compulsion. Furthermore the claim that the focus was skewed towards public safety and away from patients' rights was rejected, and the government's response stressed that the concern was about 'balancing patient and public safety with patient autonomy' (Department of Health 2005a, p.4). This response promoted the safeguards that were being proposed, including advocacy, as a means of achieving that balance, although the Joint Committee's recommendation that advocacy be available to all patients – including those not subject to the Act – was rejected. Nine months passed, and the government announced that plans for a new Bill would be abandoned in favour of amendments to the existing MH Act 1983 and, six months later, the 2006 Bill was published, receiving Royal assent in July 2007. The reasons given for this change of direction were the length and complexity of the Bill and pressures on parliamentary time (Mental Health

Alliance 2007), although the Mental Health Alliance and other grassroots activism had clearly been influential (see for example Mental Health Alliance 2005).

Critiques of the Mental Health Act 2007

The MH Act reforms have been described as an unhappy combination of legalism and safeguards, and criticised for maintaining state-sanctioned coercion (Pilgrim 2012b). The length of time to achieve the reforms and the strength of opposition are an indication of the complexity and political nature of the issues at stake, evoking Morse's description, a quarter of a century earlier, of the legalisation of commitment as 'occasion[ing] an enormous and often dismaying debate' (Morse 1982, p.55). The final resolution in the form of the MH Act 2007 has been censured for 'suppress[ing] the complexity to defend a central but disguised objective about social control' (Pilgrim 2007, p.93). Indeed, Larry Gostin (2008), a renowned Professor of Global Health Law, involved in drafting the MH Act 1983, commented:

> Historians will look back and observe that the new Mental Health Act increased the stigma of mental illness, reinforced hurtful stereotypes, de-emphasized the role of treatment as the primary justification for social action, and widened the net of compulsion in the community. It is for this reason that the World Health Organization uses the UK Act[7] as a paradigm of what not to do in mental health law reform. (p.907)

Throughout the process of reform, commentary has pointed to a shift away from rights-based thinking, evident in the initial call for radical reform, to a utilitarian approach that privileges public safety (Lepping 2007). In particular, as Gostin notes above, the absence of the principle of reciprocity is a significant shortfall, in contrast to the Mental Health (Care and Treatment) Act 2003

---

7   The MH Act 2007 covers England and Wales and not the whole of the UK.

in Scotland (Scottish Government 2005), for example. It has also been argued that without a statutory definition of risk, the MH Act 2007 enhances professional discretion, thus bringing the law into line with existing clinical practice and heralding an era of *new medicalism* (Fanning 2013). This is also evident in the broader but vague definition of mental disorder, which leaves the task of diagnosis to clinicians, so that no one needing treatment is excluded, thus favouring a duty of care over self-determination (Fistein *et al.* 2009). Furthermore, there has been concern that widening the definition of mental disorder, reducing the thresholds for treatment and extending compulsory powers to the community, in the form of supervised community treatment, would have a disproportionate impact on people from BAME communities (Vige 2009), already profoundly disadvantaged in their experience of mental health services (Keating 2007; Priebe *et al.* 2009).

These critiques have been bolstered by experience of operationalisation of the Act since 2007. This includes: widespread failure to explain people's legal rights to them to provide an opportunity to discuss them (CQC 2015a); evidence of ward cultures where control and containment are prioritised over treatment and support (CQC 2012); a perceived decline in therapeutic standards in inpatient care (CQC 2011, 2012); increasing rates of detention with consistent evidence that some groups, especially minority ethnic (BAME) communities, have higher overall detention rates (CQC 2010, 2011, 2012, 2014); and general negative experiences of care and poorer outcomes (Morgan 2012). As noted in Chapter 1, all this has occurred alongside the severest recession in living memory and significant cutbacks in NHS funding.

IMHA in the Mental Health Act 2007

The survival of IMHA as a safeguard for rights in the 2007 Act had a mixed response. Whilst widely welcomed, it was also understood to be a way of smoothing the passage of the more controversial aspects of the Act. Conversely, others viewed it as an anomaly to the general direction of the Act: 'a legalistic cuckoo' (Fanning 2014). Concerns were raised about the level of resourcing and that its introduction would unfavourably impact on the provision of other forms of advocacy that a wider constituency of people with mental health problems could access. As proposed by Barnes *et al.* (2002), the definition of IMHA in the 2007 Act describes it as a distinct form of advocacy for people detained under the legislation. The core purpose of the IMHA role is outlined in Table 4.1, and the key resources, which offer a framework for IMHA commissioning and provision, are detailed in Box 4.2.

BOX 4.2 RESOURCES FOR THE COMMISSIONING AND PROVISION OF IMHA SERVICES

The resources are:

- the MH Act 2007 supported by the Code of Practice (Department of Health 2015)

- guidance on what constitutes appropriate experience and training for IMHAs (the Mental Health Act 1983 (Independent Mental Health Advocates) (England) Regulations 2008; Standards: appropriate experience and training, Department of Health 2008)

- guidance on the access to notes by IMHAs (Department of Health 2009a) and their role in Tribunals (Ministry of Justice 2011)

- two publications providing best practice guidance: one for commissioners (National Institute for Mental Health in England (NIMHE 2008)) and one for providers (National Mental Health Development Unit (2009))

- the Health and Social Care Act 2012, which shifted responsibility for commissioning IMHA to local authorities and associated guidance

- resources from the Social Care Institute for Excellence (SCIE) and the University of Central Lancashire (2015), particularly in relation to quality indicators for a good IMHA service, 'Top 10 Tips for Commissioning IMHA', and briefings addressing inequity in IMHA provision (as listed in the Useful Resources section).

The definition of qualifying patients covered people detained under the MH Act 1983, including people on CTOs, but excluded people on emergency sections (i.e. Sections 4 and 5), thus rejecting the recommendation of the Joint Committee on the Draft Mental Health Bill 2005 that IMHA services should be available as soon as detention under the Act is being considered. Box 4.3 summarises the criteria defining eligibility for IMHA services – in other words, who the 'qualifying patient' is.

BOX 4.3 DEFINITION OF 'QUALIFYING PATIENTS'

Patients are eligible for support from an IMHA, irrespective of their age, if they are:

- detained under the Act

- liable to be detained under the Act, even if not actually detained, including those who are currently on leave of absence from hospital or absent without leave

- conditionally discharged restricted patients

- subject to guardianship

- subject to CTOs

Other patients ('informal patients') are eligible if they are:

- being considered for a treatment to which Section 57 applies (specific treatments such as psychosurgery)

- under 18 and being considered for electro-convulsive therapy (ECT) or any other treatment to which Section 58A applies.

(Source: Adapted from the Revised Code of Practice – Department of Health 2015)

Section 130A of the MH Act 1983, as amended by the MH Act 2007, requires that the appropriate authority makes arrangements for IMHAs to be available to support patients qualifying for this service in England and Wales. Post the Health and Social Care Act 2012, this means local authorities must ensure there is adequate provision of IMHA in their area. In order to fulfil their role Section 130B of the MH Act 1983 provides an IMHA with certain rights which include:

- meeting qualifying patients in private

- meeting professionals concerned with the qualifying patient's care and treatment

- accessing a patient's records, including information, which patients themselves may have no right to see, for the purpose of providing help to a qualifying patient and where the patient, or arrangements under the Court of Protection, consents. (Department of Health 2009)

To recap, the key role of an IMHA is to enable someone who is detained or subject to a CTO to: articulate their views; access information and gain a better understanding of what is happening to them; explore options, making better-informed decisions and actively engage with decisions that are being made; and participate as fully as possible in discussions and decision making relevant to them (NIMHE 2008). In working to achieve this, IMHAs should consider whether there are less restrictive treatment options and hold in mind the broader health and social outcomes for the advocacy partner (Beaupert 2009). In practice, the IMHA may provide support to enable the person to represent their own views or represent the views on behalf of the person concerned. In the case of the former, the role of the IMHA may be less visible and, as we explore in Chapter 11, may not be always appreciated by mental health professionals.

The 2007 Act makes it clear that IMHA services do not replace other advocacy and support services available to the service user and should work in conjunction with them. Equally IMHA services do not affect the individual's rights to seek legal advice and patients have the right not to use an advocate. The 2007 Act also placed a duty on mental health services to promote IMHA services to qualifying patients, although, as subsequent research has shown, this is dependent on mental health professionals understanding the role and being positively disposed to advocacy (McKeown *et al.* 2014a; Newbigging *et al.* 2012a).

The government's post-legislative scrutiny of the 2007 Act (House of Commons 2013) made a number of recommendations relating to advocacy. Reflecting a broad definition of advocacy and the need to change the relationship between people subject to compulsion and mental health professionals, these include the obligation that clinicians become the patient's advocate. This is likely to foster further confusion about the role of independent advocacy. However, the Select Committee also picked up the main strands from our research and recommendations from NICE and other bodies (Centre for Social Justice 2011; NICE 2011; Welsh Government 2011) to recommend:

- IMHA services are provided on an opt-out rather than an opt-in basis to address the difficulties qualifying patients face in accessing advocacy

- access to quality IMHA services is improved for BAME patients

- Health and Wellbeing Boards should seek specific and quantified evidence from their local commissioners to satisfy themselves that the statutory duties to provide IMHA services are being met

- the 2007 Act is amended to extend entitlement to IMHA support to all patients undergoing treatment on psychiatric wards or subject to CTOs

- the training and accountability systems for IMHAs are appropriate in the context of the role they are expected to fulfil.

Notwithstanding this, the context for the provision of IMHA services is complex. IMHAs sit at the juncture of potential conflicts of respect for autonomy and beneficence, often framed in terms of *best interests*, and the successful operation of this role requires an understanding of this positioning and competing values at stake.

IMHA: protection or promotion of rights?

Appeal to human rights is often made as a rationale for improving the social position of people experiencing mental health problems and for transforming the care and support available to enable people to get on with their lives. Human rights are universal and, therefore, being subject to compulsion and detention on the grounds of mental disorder can be argued to infringe these rights (Spandler and Calton 2009). The fact this argument has held little sway reflects the limitations of current human rights frameworks, which have been criticised for making exceptions on the basis of mental illness and assuming without question that medical treatments are necessary (Spandler and Calton 2009). Nevertheless, a human rights framework provides a useful heuristic for considering the purpose of IMHA. Vasak (1982) originally distinguished three generations of human rights, as summarised in Table 4.2, and characterised by Carpenter (2009) as liberal, egalitarian and participative.

TABLE 4.2 THREE GENERATIONS OF HUMAN RIGHTS		
Human rights	**Description**	**Examples**
First generation – political rights	Protection of individual freedom against excesses of the State; often thought of as negative rights	Right to life, freedom from abuse and degrading treatment, and freedom of speech
Second generation – economic, social and cultural rights	Underpinned by principles of human dignity, equality and anti-discrimination, these are often thought of as positive rights	Rights to food, housing, health care and welfare support
Third generation – rights to solidarity	More difficult to define and contested, covering a broad spectrum of rights relating to development, the environment and heritage	Rights to peace, self-determination, right to participation in cultural heritage, experiential rights

(Source: Adapted from Spandler and Calton 2009, Vasak 1982)

The purpose of advocacy can be construed differently within these different tiers of rights and arguably, to be effective, operates across them all. The distinction between negative and positive rights is also reflected in the UN's *Principles for the Protection of Persons with Mental Illness and for the Improvement of Mental Health Care* (Gostin 2000; Rosenthal and Rubenstein 1993) and the UN *Convention on the Rights of Persons with Disabilities* (CRPD)[8], which provide normative frameworks for national law and policies.

---

8   The CRPD was adopted by the United Nations on 13 December 2006.

IMHA services are usually framed in terms of protection of legal rights under the MH Act, that is, first generation rights, placing limits on the interference of the State on individual liberty. Examples of these are provided by a large-scale study, which recently reported on the prevalence of coercive practices on people involuntarily admitted in ten European countries, including the UK (Raboch *et al.* 2010). Such measures included physical restraint, seclusion and forced medication, and the percentage of detained patients receiving such treatment varied between 21 per cent and 59 per cent, with seclusion being used more often in the UK than other countries. A wide range of human rights infringements, both first and second generation rights, have been highlighted by successive CQC reports (CQC 2010, 2012, 2014a, 2015). These include the following:

- Pressures on beds and access to other services affecting the admission and discharge of patients mean that patients can be treated in conditions that are inappropriate and potentially represent a disproportionate interference with their human rights. For example, the rights of children and young people to dignified treatment, and to be safe and protected from harm, are adversely affected by the lack of sufficient and targeted Child and Adolescent Mental Health Services (CAMHS), leading to the admission of children to adult wards.

- Inadequate staffing ratios affect people's right to fair and dignified treatment, including a lack of staff with appropriate skills and knowledge, for example in relation to people with a learning disability, sensory impairment or from BAME communities.

- Threshold for detention being influenced by the services that are available.

- Widespread use of blanket rules, such as restrictions on access to the internet, unlimited access to activities, control over what people eat and lack of regard for cultural or religious needs.

- A lack of consistent practice when involving patients in their care decisions, such as the details of their CTO.

However, human rights issues are not always visible and will not necessarily be identified through routine monitoring visits (Russo and Rose 2013). Consultation with people having experience of detention, again in a European context, highlighted a range of human rights discrepancies including lack of interaction and general humanity of staff, receipt of unhelpful treatment, widespread reliance on psychotropic drugs, and the overall impact of compulsion on a person's life (Russo and Rose 2013). Such infringements and their concealed nature reinforce the purpose of IMHAs as providing protection for people subject to compulsion in terms of first generation rights, and with regard to second generation rights relating to the provision of health and social support that provides a range of therapeutic options.

It is clear that advocacy also has a role to play in promoting positive economic, social and cultural rights but that this may be more challenging. A mapping of the themes from focus groups with African Caribbean men identified a number of ways that mental health advocacy could bolster broader rights, including: supporting and strengthening valued identity and promoting citizenship, rather than dependence on services; securing housing, employment and access to welfare entitlements; enabling equitable access to a range of therapeutic options; and tackling racism and discrimination (Newbigging *et al.* 2007).

The extent to which IMHAs pursue this agenda, or work in partnership with other advocates to do so, clearly merits consideration. However, the strictures of the legislative framework may mean that support for this is limited. An analysis of the degree to which mental health legislation in England (and Ireland) met requirements set out by the WHO (2005), which aims to operationalise rights for people with mental health problems, found significant deficits concerning positive rights. This was particularly the case for economic and social rights, for example in relation to housing, welfare benefits and civil rights (Kelly 2011). Thus IMHAs are likely to be constrained in their role by a narrow focus on negative rights, clearly at odds with the foundational principles of advocacy.

The CRPD, underpinned by a social model of disability, is promoted as having the potential to shift the discourse from negative rights to one emphasising social rights and civic participation including rights to health, recreational and educational services, participation in community life and civil rights (Stuart 2012). There are, however, criticism of the appropriateness of treating mental health rights through a disability lens and misgivings over effectiveness of the convention, as it appears to outlaw detention on grounds of disability, which ought to render mental health legislation illegitimate (Spandler *et al.* 2015). Activists involved in the drawing up of the convention refer to supported advocacy that ensures the expressed wishes of the individual are paramount. That is, nothing is done without an individual's consent. Despite some complexities, it is argued that this is the situation with general health and that it is discriminatory to treat a person with mental impairment/psychosocial disability differently. This makes both detention and treatment without consent and the 'insanity'/diminished responsibility pleas all discriminatory (Plumb 2015).

The nature of third generation, solidarity rights is widely contested and these have not been translated into legislative frameworks in the way that first and second generation rights have. However, Creswell (2009) makes a powerful argument for experiential rights as a form of solidarity rights. He frames experiential rights as the 'right to the madness-experience' (p.236). This argument for the legitimacy of different experiences is based in the right to the *experiential whole*, compromised by the original trauma leading to service use and the subsequent institutional trauma and loss of control through encounters with the mental health system (Cresswell 2009). There are clear parallels here with Miranda Fricker's concept of epistemic injustice and the discounting of personal testimony and meaning attributed to experience (Carel and Kidd 2014; Fricker 2007). Thus advocates have a role to play in the realisation of experiential rights through supporting the expression of experience and demands that it be listened to and valued.

From the discussion of the limitations of the legislative framework and the broader conception of rights, it is evident that a narrow focus on statutory advocacy will do little to radically change the social status of service users and survivors or transform the dynamics of the mental health system. For this to be realised, advocates need to operate in a context where human rights, self-advocacy and the possibilities for recovery that validates and empowers service user experience and knowledge are actively supported. Initiatives that explicitly connect advocacy with peer support or user-led initiatives within a rights discourse will facilitate this. Box 4.4 provides one such example where the advocate recognises the importance of ensuring a better understanding of rights amongst service users, capitalising on the potential to promote empowerment. Equally, it is evident that recovery-oriented services that include peer-led initiatives, such as Wellness Recovery Action Planning (WRAP), increase people's capacity to self-advocate (Jonikas *et al.* 2013), thus potentially reducing need for IMHA services.

BOX 4.4 *MAD ABOUT RIGHTS*

As an advocate for a consumer/psychiatric survivor advocacy group – the Empowerment Council – the primary focus of my work is to address systemic inequalities in a large urban psychiatric hospital in Toronto, Canada. While there have been improvements and more transparency in the psychiatric system over the years, there remain many urgent and new challenges. In order for service users to have more agency in their own health care, a continued effort to create spaces and share education in an accessible, bold and forthright manner on the importance of rights is essential.

What is *Mad about Rights*?

Mad about Rights is an eight-week primer on mental health rights accessed by detained persons directly within the hospital. It was developed to bridge the gap between medico-legal texts and service user personal experiences in the mental health system. The overall goal of the sessions is to teach service user students about: the *Canadian Charter of Rights and Freedoms*; important mental health legal cases; courts and Tribunals; the differences between the Health Care Consent Act and Substitute Decisions Act; the ex-patient movement; and finally some reflexivity skills informed by personal experiences with access to rights/advocacy.

Students are introduced to national and local frameworks for rights and read seminal articles about consumers/survivors such as by Geoff Reaume, Judi Chamberlin and Persimmon Blackbridge; explore how race, gender and class intersect with narratives of madness; and work through complex concepts such as oppression, marginalisation and empowerment so that they can appreciate the opportunities and limitations of these terms and the implications in their own lives. Privilege and power are also analysed by reading essays, poems or first-person writings from psychiatric survivors. By week five, students begin to engage in discussion about their own social locations and identities and the implications of variations depending on access to power or privilege.

Why is *Mad about Rights* important?

Service users who sign up for the *Mad about Rights* primer are exposed to a range of ideas and concepts that teach them about their rights in the system and also allow them to share stories and experiences in a small group. Service users are always keen to learn more about law and advocacy, and at times they have described this as being beneficial towards goals of employment, particularly if they want peer support jobs. It helps with the isolation that some service users feel while staying in the hospital and assists in making school and learning a less scary prospect. Until psychiatrists and other clinicians acknowledge and comply with the law as it pertains to mental health service users, then the work of education will continue to rest on all of us to facilitate opportunities for more consciousness raising and inclusion of their voice.

Lucy Costa

The challenge, therefore, is to develop the social and intellectual capital of local actors in the mental health system in respect of recovery and rights, and advocacy organisations have a key role in this respect, alongside service user organisations.

Conclusions

The conception of rights within the MH Act has implications for the provision of IMHA services and how they operate on a day-to-day basis, as well as shaping the context within which both advocates and people subject to compulsion are situated. Our analysis of the legal context begs certain questions as to the purpose and role of IMHAs, and the extent to which their focus is restricted to negative rights or more ambitiously oriented to the realisation of social, economic, cultural and experiential rights. Whilst the MH Act might appear opposed to a wider focus, the foundational principles of advocacy would certainly support it, locating IMHA within a broader concern for human rights as opposed to a constricted interpretation of the role as merely a legalistic measure. Clearly, values play a central role in the interpretation of human rights in the mental health context, reflecting the complexities of human needs and capabilities, as well as prevailing social and political circumstances (Kelly 2011). This has implications for the training and support of IMHAs, as well as their relationships with mental health professionals, which will ultimately impact on the outcomes and future life chances of people subject to compulsion.

REFLECTIVE EXERCISES

1. Identify from the discussion in this chapter at least two different ways in which advocacy is framed in relation to the promotion and protection of human rights. How do these different ideas affect the potential role of independent advocates?

2. Consider the function of IMHA under the MH Act and the notion of self-determination. Does the discussion highlight any challenges for promoting the human rights of people subject to compulsion?

3. IMHA as framed in the MH Act seeks to address powerlessness and inequity. How can IMHAs support the self-determination of people subject to compulsion?

4. List at least two ways in which the MH Act (a) promotes recovery and service user-identified goals and (b) does NOT promote this. What do your lists tell you about the extent to which the MH Act is able to promote recovery?

Chapter 5

'MY RIGHTS TO MY VOICE'

Service User Experiences of Compulsion

Introduction

The number of people detained under the MH Act has been rising since the mid-1990s, and in 2013/14 the MH Act was used 53,176 times to detain people in hospital for longer than 72 hours, a 5 per cent increase in numbers since 2012/13 and a 30 per cent increase since 2003/04 (CQC 2015a, p.35). Furthermore, despite opposition and widespread concerns, the use of CTOs has continued to rise and exceed predictions (Stroud, Doughty and Banks 2013). Detention under the MH Act, variously referred to as 'being sectioned' or involuntary hospital admission and treatment, has a profound personal and social impact, and in this chapter we explore experiences of these measures from a service user perspective. Whilst we focus on people who are formally detained and eligible for IMHA, it is evident that voluntary patients can also experience coercion to comply with treatment and detention (34% in Katsakou *et al.*'s 2011 study). Indeed the 'de facto' detention of informal patients, whose liberty to leave hospital is compromised because they are unaware of their rights or fearful that they might be sectioned should they try, is a longstanding concern.[1]

This chapter focuses on service user narratives within a range of studies to explore the first-hand experiences of compulsion under mental health law, using quotations from participants in various studies and our own research to illustrate key themes. We explore experiences at different stages of the process of admission, treatment and discharge, summarising the common

---

1   See for example Hansard for 17 January 2007, pt0013.

themes that IMHAs are likely to encounter, and which influence views of this experience. However, we start by reflecting on the nature of studies of compulsion, drawing attention to some of the methodological issues that have been highlighted.

Studies of compulsion

Rating scales have been widely used to understand the impact of coercion, and whilst these enable comparisons to be made, they are a poor method for eliciting the diversity and depth of people's experiences (Russo and Wallcraft 2011). The credibility, trustworthiness and transferability of some research findings in relation to compulsion has also been called into question. For example, a review of five studies of involuntary hospital admission and treatment identified a range of methodological weaknesses, including small sample size, minimal details of the analytical steps, and no discussion of researcher bias (Katsakou and Priebe 2007). Methods of recruiting participants to such studies can also be problematic, relying on convenience sampling (Katsakou and Priebe 2007) or on staff selection of participants, making their own judgments about 'suitable' research participants. Furthermore, people from particular groups are not included or the data not analysed in terms of the demographic characteristics of the participants, thus limiting our understanding of the impact of compulsion on diverse groups.

A more penetrating criticism highlights 'the problematic proximity between compulsory treatment and its psychiatric research', with research largely being undertaken by clinicians who shape the questions to be asked and may be involved as interviewers as well as providing care (Russo and Wallcraft 2011, p.221) – thus calling into question findings that point to high levels of satisfaction with compulsion (Russo and Wallcraft 2011). Arguably, the very nature of compulsion requires that research is either service user led or service user controlled, or at the very least co-produced with people with lived experience of compulsion.

User or survivor involvement in research, either through co-production or through user-controlled projects, is a relatively recent development (Faulkner and Thomas 2002; Turner and Beresford 2005), such that the evidence about the impact or process of involvement of service users in health and social care research is currently limited (Brett *et al.* 2014; Caldon *et al.* 2010). A potential strength is that service user or peer researchers place a different emphasis in their approach to inquiry than traditional researchers, emphasising experiences, feelings and the reality of daily living over processes and biomedical approaches (Gillard *et al.* 2010). Furthermore, participants interviewed by service user researchers have described the benefits of comradeship, as well as some concerns around insecurity (Bengtsson-Tops and Svensson 2010). However, possibly the main benefits are the potential to generate new knowledge about the experience of detention by people who have been detained, shaping the research focus and interpretive analysis (Gillard *et al.* 2010; Rose 2009).

In this chapter, we therefore draw heavily on our research, including past studies of compulsion, as this has been undertaken in partnership with service users, including those with lived experience of compulsion. Service users were involved throughout the research, which has deployed qualitative methods to capture the richness and diversity of people's experience (Newbigging *et al.* 2012a; Ridley 2014; Ridley and Hunter 2013).

Experience of detention

By definition, detention under the MH Act is against the person's will and, consequently, it could be anticipated that the majority of accounts would be negative; most people do not like being forced to do something they don't want or prevented from doing something they do. However, studies of subjective experiences of compulsion reveal a mixed picture, with experiences of compulsion as unhelpful, profoundly disempowering and humiliating contrasted with some experiences that are supportive and helpful (Johansson and Lundman 2002; Ridley 2014; Ridley and Hunter 2013). There are also contradictory responses to detention reported, with individuals 'simultaneously accepting and resisting the orders' (Canvin, Bartlett and Pinfold 2002, p.361). Katsakou and Priebe (2007) observe, however, that, without more details from the primary data, it can be difficult with some studies to discern whether mixed views of detention were from different people or whether the same individual's views changed over time.

One study, involving peer researchers, used interviews with a cohort of service users at two stages ten months apart to explore their views of new mental health legislation in a Scottish context. Coercion was found to be universally unwelcome and associated with overwhelming feelings of powerlessness and loss (Ridley 2014). However, half of the people in the second stage interview reflected that 'compulsion had been the "right thing" for them at the time, a "necessary evil"' (Ridley and Hunter 2013, p.513). This finding is reflected in other studies, which have implied incongruence between a patient's legal status and their experience of coercion, suggesting that between a fifth and three-quarters of detained patients appreciate the need for hospitalisation, while half of voluntary patients experience their care as coercive (Hiday et al. 1997; O'Donoghue et al. 2010).

Some of the reported contradictions may be due to shortcomings in study design or method. For example, in the study by O'Donoghue et al. (2010) noted earlier, 72 per cent of the participants thought their detention had been necessary. However, the interviews were conducted by psychiatrists in the period after detention and before discharge from hospital, when the interviewees' treatment was still reliant on the opinions of clinicians. This specific timing is thus likely to have an effect on which opinions they might feel able to express. This was not the case in the study by Ridley and Hunter (2013), however, which was carried out in partnership with nine service users and consideration given to strategies to redress the power imbalances between interviewers and interviewees.

An individual person may express a range of opinions about their detention at different points along their pathway through mental health services. The extent to which these are understood is debatable, with some researchers suggesting that reports of negative experiences of compulsion reflect an individual's mental health status such that all staff activity, no matter how caring, will be interpreted as intrusive, coercive and unwelcome[2] (Wyder, Bland and Crompton 2013), thus reinforcing the need for service user-led research in this area. Individual journeys involving detention may cover many years: some people may be admitted once, for a relatively short time, while others may be on a ward for many months or years. Some people are re-admitted several times, or they may be discharged on a CTO which allows for compulsory re-admission to a ward and requires compliance with treatment, usually medication. Experiences of detention are likely to be influenced by where people are on this journey. However, this is not to suggest that such a journey is linear; rather, it is more complex, and in periods of 'non-compulsion' people may experience less than stable circumstances (Ridley 2014).

Admission under the MH Act

The period leading up to an assessment under the MH Act is rarely included in studies, but reports from service users and carers suggest that this is a crucial and traumatic point in time when people are extremely distressed. Healthtalk has several short videos of people describing the circumstances leading up to admission, the process and first impressions of acute in-patient wards.[3] Service users and carers can feel that if they had been

---

2   An interesting study in the different context of midwifery suggests that women giving birth are likely to view traumatic experiences differently depending upon the perceived kindness of the midwife. Effectively, the mothers were less upset by a greater degree of (objectively) traumatic experience if it appeared to be enacted with care, but could be exceedingly upset by seemingly lesser trauma if accompanied by an uncaring midwife (Thomson and Downe 2010).

3   See for example www.healthtalk.org/peoples-experiences/mental-health/experiences-psychosis/hospital-treatment-and-compulsory-care (accessed on 26 January 2015).

listened to earlier and prompt care and support offered when requested, detention could have been avoided:

> I was phoning his doctor a lot of times. I phoned the police and the police used to say 'until he does something we can't intervene' and the doctor would say 'if you're worried about him phone the police' and this went on and on and he got worse. (Mother quoted in Ridley *et al.* 2014, p.28)

This is further emphasised in recent reports on crisis care, which highlight variations in the help, care and support available to people in a crisis (CQC 2015b). Service user and carers emphasise the importance of an appropriate and timely response from services to requests for help.

> The support I need to ward off a full-blown crisis is fairly simple and straightforward and definitely cheaper than hospitalisation. I need emotional space to talk to someone outside of my everyday life about what is going on for me... I can identify what does help, but at time of crisis lose sight of these things and literally just need someone to be calm, available to connect to and to remind me of these strategies. (Mind 2011, p.12)

People describe their need for accessible, safe places that are open at all hours, where they are protected from harming themselves, and where they feel that someone cares about them and will support them. Many people have this expectation of acute wards in hospital (Mind 2011). However, it is now common for in-patient environments to be locked and custodial, contrasting with the open and trusting safe space requested by people as they fall into a crisis. A lack of beds also means that accessing care can be challenging even when detention is being considered, leaving many people, including children, spending nights in a police cell because of a lack of beds (Centre for Social Justice 2011).[4] It may

---

4   Some 263 children were in custody in 2014–15 (House of Commons Health Committee – Children and Adolescents' Mental Health and Child and Adolescent Mental Health Services, 3rd report of session 2014–15 p.55).

also result in people being admitted to hospital at considerable distance from their home, making contact and support from family and friends difficult, potentially compounding feelings of isolation and distress and contravening the right to family life.

Involuntary admission can be a life-changing experience with an impact on self-esteem, health, relationships, employment and community life (Sibitz *et al.* 2011) and represent an unwanted disruption to everyday life (Katsakou *et al.* 2012). Some people with previous experience of detention, however, may see use of the MH Act as the only realistic way to obtain the support they need:

> On the whole, I was glad I was in hospital because I knew if I wasn't I'd have cut myself to bits at home so I knew I was in the right place. (IMHA partner, psychiatric intensive care unit, quoted in Newbigging *et al.* 2012a, p.59)

> I asked for the CPN [community psychiatric nurse] to section me before I got violent and everything like this. (Non-IMHA user, acute ward, quoted in Newbigging *et al.* 2012a, p.58)

For many, however, it was related to a lack of viable alternatives: 'It feels like I literally have to have one foot off the bridge before I can access services' (interviewee quoted in Mind 2011, p.18). Another person (quoted in Ridley and Hunter 2013, p.513) stated:

> Well it could stop me from getting into any more trouble than I already got myself into. Somehow, it kept me stable…there would have been better ways of dealing with it, much better ways of dealing with it than hospitalisation.

Given the circumstances leading up to hospital admission for some people, the police may be involved, which can be hard to understand for people who see law enforcement as separate to health care. In instances involving the police, the level of force used had felt excessive:

> They rang up the doctors, the doctors rang the police, they came to collect me from the train station. I was brought in

here in a police van. I wasn't a criminal, I wasn't dangerous, I wasn't hitting anybody or being a threat. (IMHA partner, acute ward, quoted in Newbigging *et al.* 2012a, p.60)

The process of admission to hospital can be retraumatising, evoking earlier experiences of coercion or abuse (Sapey 2013), and be a disturbing time for the whole family as well as the individual. None of the studies focusing on experiences of detention mentioned the potential use of advocacy or peer support during the admission process to reduce the consequent feelings of powerlessness, isolation and shock.

I will not forget when the door shut and we had to leave him in the psychiatric ward. It was a horrible feeling…I was completely in shock. (Mother quoted in Gerson *et al.* 2009, p.813).

And then he [the physician] just, he was so…rude, he flared up and 'Well now you will be admitted to involuntary care' and that was all and then he left the room. And then I just sat there totally taken aback. (Patient quoted in Johansson and Lundman 2002, p.643)

It can be seen from these accounts that the process of admission can be bewildering, disempowering and frightening, resonating with Kris Chastey's account in the Foreword. It is also clear that in some instances people have unsuccessfully sought help prior to detention and its inaccessibility compounds feelings of being misunderstood and frustration, and fuels potential resistance to admission. Furthermore, people may not understand what is happening to them or, even when they are clear about the measures being applied, may be vague about the expected duration of their detention or their rights (Ridley 2014). People subject to compulsion might also be acutely distressed or experiencing the sedating effects of medication, so may not comprehend why they are in hospital. Whilst providing information is critical, the way in which this is done needs to be thoughtful and take account of the person's capacity for information at the time of admission, so that information about rights is provided in the most effective manner.

On the ward

People who use services are very clear about the kind of support they would find helpful in a crisis, including prompt access to a calm place where they can talk to someone in a safe environment. Key attitudes and values required from staff include respect, warmth, compassion and understanding (Mind 2011, p.12). Specific suggestions of helpful services include user-led services such as crisis houses and peer support (James 2010; O'Hagan 2011) and alternative forms of professionally led discussion such as Open Dialogue (Seikkula, Alakare and Aaltonen 2011). Other potentially beneficial suggestions include advance directives, which have been shown to reduce compulsory admissions, although difficulties in implementation mean that, in practice, few people are aware of them (Henderson *et al.* 2004; Jankovic, Richards and Priebe 2010).

Themes that have emerged from qualitative studies of detention emphasise the need for caring and supportive relationships (Gault 2009; Gilburt, Rose and Slade 2008; Hughes, Hayward and Finlay 2009); participation in decision making (Katsakou and Priebe 2007); and safe emotional environments offering respectful care (Andreasson and Skärsäter 2012; Gilburt *et al.* 2008). While there are good services that provide helpful support and are recovery focused (Papoulias *et al.* 2014), ward environments are often frightening places such that people in crisis describe them as traumatising and impersonal settings, which they would want to avoid (Mind 2011). People who have a history of admissions may have difficult memories of ward care which override any improvements that have been made by recent initiatives such as Star Wards (2008) or Accreditation for Inpatient Mental Health Services (AIMS) by the Royal College of Psychiatrists (2014).

Guidance highlights the role of a therapeutic environment, including gender-specific sleeping and bathing facilities, access to fresh air, quiet space and a range of activities (Khan and Daw 2011), but even these basic standards may not be met – a cause of concern to families as much as people on wards or inspecting bodies such as the CQC: 'Carers require that the ward environment adheres to the basic standards such as good toilet facilities and privacy. Carers feel upset when the inpatient environment is unkempt' (carer quoted in Askey *et al.* 2009, p.320).

Ward routines may be helpful for some in providing a safe and predictable space, but can be a source of frustration for people who have been experiencing a more chaotic life. Regular meals and a fixed sleeping regimen can be unfamiliar for many patients, while others may have additional difficulties around withdrawing from substances or alcohol. There is often limited access to activities which would potentially be a welcomed distraction (Ridley and Hunter 2013). Furthermore, access to family and friends can be restricted, either as visitors to a ward or through social media and use of mobile phones. Safety procedures, such as removing furniture or belongings, can be seen as punitive. The application of 'blanket rules' to all service users curbs choice and may breach human rights (CQC 2014).

Disinhibited, threatening or aggressive behaviour from other patients results in many people feeling unsafe on wards (Wood and Pistrang 2004). Examples of bullying and racist, sexist or homophobic insults or attacks, including physical or sexual assaults, have been variously reported:

> Such common terms as 'black bastard' [and] 'nxxxxx' would be common place in daily confrontations as well as physical assault, at times quite violent physical assault. It made me very insecure… A blind eye was taken and in fact on one occasion where there was quite clear racial intimidation present, a nurse said 'not in here, take that outside, sort yourselves out outside'. (In-patient from a BAME background quoted in Ridley 2014, p.190)

This quote illustrates the potential for complicity by staff and how the handling of such incidents will influence the service user perceptions of staff and safety of the ward environment.

Wider, overarching issues such as institutional racism, have long been remarked upon, and were brought to a sharp focus as a consequence of the enquiry into the death of David Bennett.[5] As his sister commented, 'He told me he was racially abused and that he was taunted and was not prepared to tolerate it' (NSC NHS Strategic Health Authority 2003, p.8).

However, personal experiences may remain hidden from institutional observers, and organisational and professional norms that shape practice may go unquestioned. For example, the specific needs of people from BAME communities can be typically construed in terms of language and interpreting services without consideration of broader cultural or personalised needs (Newbigging *et al.* 2012a). Similarly, the gender-specific needs of women, men and transgender people can also be unappreciated, despite the introduction of gender-specific in-patient facilities. People with learning disabilities can receive poor care, as highlighted in the extreme by the Winterbourne View scandal (Department of Health 2012) and inspections of other establishments.[6]

An important aspect of ward culture and atmosphere is the existence of comradely support between fellow service users, and the extent to which this builds a sense of 'community' that is helpful and sustaining:

> The good things are meeting people that have got mental health problems. I've made a few friends…and we'll all meet up now and again sometimes here or at P's flat, and it's good because you can relate with each other and you're going through the same experiences. (In-patient quoted in Ridley 2014, p.191)

---

5   David (Rocky) Bennett was an African Caribbean man with a history of schizophrenia, who was detained in a medium secure unit. He died following restraint by staff.

6   As a result, campaigners are seeking to remove people with learning disabilities and autistic spectrum from the jurisdiction of the MH Act. http://lbbill.wordpress.com, 2014.

The importance of being seen as a person, with past experience, capabilities and shared humanity being respected, cannot be underestimated. Findings from a literature review that looked at patients' experiences of the quality of care during compulsory admission indicated that to the extent to which people felt listened to, or otherwise, was the defining feature of their experiences (Hooff and Goossensen 2013). However, even when there were increased opportunities for involvement, it did not necessarily result in people's views being taken into account (Ridley and Hunter 2013). Staff dispositions can reportedly change depending on the context in which encounters take place, and the ward environment and legal status of service users can contribute to a sense of invalidation:

> Last year I ended up in hospital. On the Monday and Tuesday I was [delivering] training. Everybody was very attentive and respectful and wanted to hear what I had to say. On the Wednesday I got sectioned and by evening I was in the ward where nobody had the slightest interest in what I was saying or what my views were and it was all down to my pathology. And I was suddenly a total non-entity and it was really weird how suddenly you could overnight just change...be treated so differently. (Service user consultant quoted in Kalathil 2011, p.26)

Consequently, while people anticipate that a hospital will offer safety and comfort in a caring environment, this may not be the experience of people admitted to psychiatric wards, particularly for those detained against their will.

Compulsory treatment

The importance of choice is consistently emphasised by service users, and this applies as much, if not more, to compulsory detention and treatment and will have a bearing on individual self-esteem and recovery (Valenti *et al.* 2014): 'It's a different feeling, you know, when you're doing something because you want to rather than feeling that you're still struggling against something that you may never get off' (IMHA partner, acute ward, quoted in Newbigging *et al.* 2012a, p.63). Once admitted, a person may have little say in their treatment, which can include use of forced medication, physical restraint and seclusion, in turn resulting in problematic interactions with staff, which may spark incidents of aggression (Duxbury and Whittington 2005). The treatment options for people detained under the Act are typically limited or simply equate to drug therapies (CQC 2014; Ridley and Hunter 2013), leaving many feeling they have few options (Roberts *et al.* 2008). People who are detained are more likely to refuse medication than voluntary patients (Owiti and Bowers 2010). There are many reasons for not wanting to take medication, including ambivalent or positive disposition towards experiences deemed as symptoms, such as hearing voices for example, or concerns that the medical remedy effectively means a return to a miserable everyday life (Roberts *et al.* 2008). There may also be unwanted side effects which add to distress rather than facilitating recovery:

> They gave me medication where I couldn't breathe [...] I couldn't sit down [...] and I felt drowsy, tired. Not the kind of drowsy where you think, oh, I'll have a good night's sleep. It's the kind of drowsy where you think, oh, I'm going to die in a minute. (Participant quoted in Hughes *et al.* 2009, p.157)

> I couldn't talk, my mouth was locking, my mouth was like twisting, it really hurt [...] And I couldn't talk to let them know what was wrong. (Participant quoted in Hughes *et al.* 2009, p.157)

Consequently, while staff may feel that drug treatments are clinically necessary and in the patient's 'best interests', service users may fundamentally disagree (Haglund, von Knorring and von Essen 2003). The conflicts that arise because of a refusal of medication may then initiate actions resulting in forced administration of medication. Despite the policy emphasis on concordance, a lack of negotiation between people who are detained and mental health professionals is sadly evident:

> I used to plead with them and plead with them (tearful), please don't give me that [medication]. And of course that used to make me more crazy, because I didn't know where to turn, I didn't know what to do (crying) […] the more bad I was, the more I knew I was going to be medicated, so the more crazy I got, because I was terrified. (Participant quoted in Hughes *et al.* 2009, p.157)

There may be little communication or explanation, or opportunity for others to intervene or offer support.

> It made no difference that I'd stepped out of a meeting with the IMHA to get a letter from my bedroom she'd asked to see. They came in as I sat on the floor, document wallet in hand, surrounded by papers. They did it to me there, then walked off chatting, leaving me to wander back to the IMHA, dishevelled and dazed. (@Sectioned_ 2014a)

Without negotiation, attempts to medicate may be resisted, leading to the use of restraint:

> I become aggressive when they use violence, it's an encroachment when they don't say anything but just catch hold of you and drag you to the bed and give the injection with force and a lot of people are holding you. They didn't have to use violence… They didn't need a whole army from two wards. (Patient quoted in Johansson and Lundman 2002, p.643)

Such treatment can then result in people behaving in ways that are out of character for them, such that their resulting behaviour is considered to be further evidence of mental disorder: 'I did say to them, if you treat me like an animal, then I'll act like an animal. Why are you doing this, to me? You know, because I was acting, totally out of character' ('Sarah' quoted in Hughes *et al.* 2009, p.157). Forced treatment may then continue to be repeated regularly without explanation, leaving the person with a lasting trauma:

I recall time and again being left face down, underwear and trousers askew, in sheets covered in bootprints on a bed pushed out from the wall, empty antiseptic wipe packets on the floor. I'd be left shocked, terrorised, humiliated, confused, frightened, to clear up my bedspace, somehow get hold of clean sheets and somehow work out how to, well, be on the ward again. (@Sectioned_ 2014b)

Opposing views about the most appropriate treatment, coupled with the power imbalance between service users and mental health professionals, can impede the growth of a trusting relationship. For some time, however, critical commentators have been urging more democratic forms of shared decision making regarding medication, largely with a view to improving concordance, involving negotiation between the service user and clinical team (Gray, Wykes and Gournay 2002; Piatkowska and Farnill 1992). Ridley and Hunter (2013), for example, noted some instances where a change of medication had been negotiated, reflecting some progress towards more concordant approaches. One study of the degree to which psychiatrists put pressure on service users to agree to treatment plans or prescriptions that are seen to be in their best interests distinguished three types of interaction between prescribing psychiatrists and service users (Quirk *et al.* 2012). These encounters were described as open (where decision making was freely negotiated with full participation of the service user); or they were largely directed by the psychiatrist, with the service user cooperating, but being gently led towards the position preferred by the psychiatrist in the first place; or they were pressured (the psychiatrist more or less badgers the service user into accepting the practitioner point of view). It is unclear, but likely, that the legislative framework of compulsion influences psychiatric practice negatively and away from shared decision making, raising interesting questions about the role of advocacy in promoting service user preferences.

Experiences of restraint and seclusion

Common coercive practices to which service users may be subject include physical restraint, seclusion and chemical restraint. These in turn may increase the level of verbal threats, physical assault and damage to the environment. A link has been identified between staff characteristics such as authoritarian behaviour and consequent aggression and violence from patients (Duxbury 2011). As noted earlier, the initial process of detaining people against their wishes may involve a level of force, which can feel excessive and may lead to physical injury. This may be re-enacted once on the ward:

> I was hurt when they restrained me and they put your arms behind you and push your head down and take you to a quiet room, I was hurt and I'm still hurt now, I'm receiving physiotherapy for it. (IMHA partner, acute ward, quoted in Newbigging *et al.* 2012a, p.61)

As one participant in research commissioned by Mind (2011) commented: 'Go in for recovery…come out injured' (p.25). Physical restraint can be humiliating, painful and potentially life threatening, with concern over a number of restraint-related deaths (Independent Advisory Panel on Deaths in Custody 2014 Strategic Health Authority 2003).[7] It can be traumatic to witness and sends out specific messages around required behaviour to other people on the ward. The *Count Me In* census in 2010 found that about 12 per cent of patients had experienced one or more episodes of physical restraint, but did not register how many patients had witnessed such events (CQC 2011). Mixed feelings about seclusion are reported, with some people feeling anger and fear, but others a sense of safety (Kontio *et al.* 2012).

---

7   There were 282 deaths of people detained under the MH Act in 2013 and 341 in 2012, an increase of nearly 20 per cent on the previous year. The majority of these were deaths from natural causes but, in 2012, there were 14 deaths where restraint was identified as either a contributory or direct cause of death or happened in the seven days preceding the death.

A not unusual experience can be the contrast between the frightening chaos of a forced removal to seclusion, with the terrifying sense of isolation once there: 'Especially these heavy doors and...they slam shut behind you and...I have never experienced such loneliness' (R7 quoted in Hoekstra *et al.* 2004, p.280). Meehan, Bergen and Fjeldsoe (2004) found that while all staff in their study believed in the calming and positive effect of seclusion, two-thirds of patients believed it never made them feel better. Such experiences of coercion impact on the way that staff are viewed:

> I'm too frightened of them... I'm terrified of them, terrified. I'm terrified of being jabbed in the bottom or being put in their cooler. So I'm too frightened of them, terrible state of affairs. And this is supposed to be a hospital. (Geraldine quoted in Wood and Pistrang 2004, p.23)

This is a reality that is also acknowledged by some staff:

> It must feel like being attacked. Although we're all trained to do that [restraint] in a harmless way, without inflicting any pain...it just must be terrifying. I wouldn't like to be on the receiving end at all. (Naomi quoted in Wood and Pistrang 2004, p.24)

In addition to these coercive experiences, there may be other physical restrictions placed on individuals such that the everyday routine of a ward can feel oppressive and constraining. Wards are frequently locked and people who are detained may need to wait for staff to accompany them off the ward, even when this is just to access outdoor space such as gardens. Legislation that prevents smoking indoors, while helpful for health promotion, can be challenging for people unable to exercise choice about accessing outdoor spaces. Waiting for staff to accompany them outside can be a source of frustration on busy wards where staff need to prioritise other emergencies. Patients have suggested it would be helpful to speak to an independent person about their experiences of coercion: 'I want to talk with an outside evaluator, patient representative (ombudsman, chaplain) about my thoughts and especially after seclusion/restraint' (Kontio *et al.* 2012, p.20).

Discharge from detention

The prospect of relaxing applied restrictions or discharge from detention can feel remote, compounded by a sense that one's voice is not heard. In circumstances where service users feel their initial symptoms have gone, they may feel they will not be believed and forced to remain on a ward with their detention prolonged. Consequently, service users can feel pressured to behave passively and obey rules, although they can experience care and treatment regimens as prison-like and worthy of resisting: 'Being a good patient leads to getting my freedom back (i.e. escaping the ward)' (service user quoted in Gault 2009, p.509); and:

> Something I, and many others, do is to 'fake it to make it' or 'believe it to achieve it', meaning that I'd behave as if I was better than I actually felt in order to have a section lifted and thus 'escape'. (Service user (J.W.) quoted in Roberts *et al.* 2008, p.175)

Conditions of discharge onto a CTO include a requirement to accept medication, to see specific staff, or to live at a specified location. Where a person disagrees, this may be interpreted by mental health staff as threatening or risky. Service users often lack awareness about the power of the CTO and can be ambivalent about its use (Stroud *et al.* 2013). A range of service user perspectives on CTOs vary, described as 'a draconian measure' and alternatively 'a comforting safety net' (Ridley 2014, p.191), whilst some people emphasise the greater freedom allowed compared with hospital-based detention, while ensuring access to care (Gibbs *et al.* 2005).

Whilst the conditions of discharge are important, if the circumstances to which people are returning are unchanged, any benefits from compulsory detention and treatment are likely to be short lived. Furthermore, if the experience of hospitalisation and discharge has been wholly negative, the situation may be even more disheartening. The importance of family, friends, meaningful employment, a decent income, a safe place to live and freedom from abuse have consistently been implicated as necessary for mental health. The extent to which these are properly considered is debatable given the tendency to focus on medication and to pay less attention to non-clinical, social, psychological and other support required for enabling recovery and a good quality of life (Ridley 2014).

The longer-term impact of compulsion

'Being sectioned' can not only disrupt people's lives but may have a lasting legacy in the form of stigma. It can therefore compound social disadvantage, discrimination and inequalities for people experiencing mental health problems (Russo and Wallcraft 2011). For example, large numbers of people lose their jobs or take a significant time to return to work following admission to acute care (Blank et al. 2008). Similarly, people can find themselves increasingly isolated or homeless (Tulloch, Fearon and David 2012). Furthermore, in attempting to recover these aspects of their life, people are likely to encounter negative stereotypes and stigma that reduce their chances of doing so and ultimately undermine self-esteem and identity. Thus, the experience of powerlessness persists beyond the immediate period of admission, having consequences for individual mental health and potentially shaping attitudes to future help seeking.

Autonomy, participation, care and recovery

Feelings of powerlessness and lack of control are almost a universal experience of compulsion, despite the great majority of people believing their mental health was poor prior to admission (Katsakou et al. 2012). A substantial proportion of people regard hospital admission as neither justified nor beneficial (Katsakou and Priebe 2007).

The research literature identifies common themes and experiences raised by people who have been subject to compulsion. First, experiences of violation of autonomy are commonly mentioned and these include rights being taken away, lack of options and meaningful voice in treatment, an absence of information on treatment, views being ignored, inflexible ward regimes and not being allowed to be responsible for themselves, in addition to the physical violations highlighted earlier (Katsakou and Priebe 2007; Wyder et al. 2013). Those who thought less coercive measures would have been more appropriate experienced detention as an unjust infringement of their autonomy (Katsakou et al. 2012), whereas this was less likely for people who were informed about their rights (Katsakou and Priebe 2007), and for those moved to less restrictive options as quickly as possible (Wyder et al. 2013).

Second, and related to the first, is the issue of participation in decision making and effective influence on treatment decisions. Many people felt the need for help and support, but not having their issues heard or views on treatment options taken into account contributed to feelings that rights had been taken away and exposed the power imbalance between them and professional staff (Wyder et al. 2013). Conversely, those people given opportunities to participate in their own care and treatment reported feeling more empowered and more likely to accept the professionally defined need for compulsory treatment (Wyder et al. 2013).

Third, the importance of respectful therapeutic relationships with professionals and communicative competence are recurrent themes, as opposed to a narrow focus on compliance with treatment regimes (Gault 2009; McKeown et al. 2014c; Ridley 2014). In particular, the feeling of being cared for, that you are being looked after, that people have an interest in you, take time with you and are committed to your recovery, are essential in fulfilling the expectation that hospital will be a place of safety (Katsakou and Priebe 2007).

The ward culture plays an important role in determining the therapeutic milieu for detained patients. This clearly extends beyond direct interactions with staff to the quality of relationships with friends and family and camaraderie with other patients.

A lack of activity, boredom, being forced to live with seriously unwell people in cramped and mixed wards and poor staff attitudes were associated with negative perceptions of detention (Ridley and Hunter 2013).

Nonetheless, it is good relationships with staff that are central, as 'being seen and treated as a fellow human being (shared humanity), being respected and heard', and feeling safe are repeatedly identified as contributing to more positive experiences of detention (Wyder *et al.* 2013, p.578). Unsurprisingly these are what service users also identify as important characteristics of IMHAs, as explored in Chapter 9. Conversely, people who experienced a more punitive dynamic with staff were more likely to describe detention as detrimental to their recovery, reinforcing a negative self-image and making it harder to incorporate the experience and come to terms with the emotional impact of detention and the disruption to their lives.

Finally, and linked to all of the above, is the extent to which independent mental health advocacy needs to be underpinned by a commitment to minimize the harms of compulsory detention and treatment. 'Recovery', an idea borrowed from the service user movement, was defined for mental health services by William Anthony (1993) over 20 years ago (see Box 5.1), and more recently framed in progressive terms of hope, courage, control and opportunities (Repper 2011):

> It is by having the **hope** that things can get better, and the courage to move on, that we can learn about what works for us and gain **control** of our difficulties, so that we can pursue **opportunities** and live a meaningful and fulfilling life.

BOX 5.1 DEFINITION OF RECOVERY

Recovery is a deeply personal, unique process of changing one's attitudes, values, feelings, goals, skills and/or roles. It is a way of living a satisfying, hopeful and contributing life even with limitations caused by the illness. Recovery involves the development of new meaning and purpose in one's life as one grows beyond the catastrophic effects of mental illness.

Recovery from mental illness involves much more than recovery from the illness itself. People with mental illness may have to recover from the stigma they have incorporated into their very being; from the iatrogenic effects of treatment settings; from lack of recent opportunities for self-determination; from the negative side effects of unemployment; and from crushed dreams. Recovery is often a complex, time-consuming process.

(Source: Anthony 1993, p.527)

Within such a paradigm,[8] if the experience of mental health services is to be transformed, every interaction needs to be recovery focused and based on a partnership between 'experts' (people with lived experience, carers and mental health professionals). Authentically recovery-orientated services provide for increasing personalisation and choice to enable people to meet their goals, and enjoy a 'life beyond illness'.[9] Clearly detaining people against their will runs counter to the principles of recovery and reinforces stigma and exclusion (Perkins and Repper 2014). However, as subsequent chapters show, IMHAs need to promote a recovery-focused approach through enabling shared decision making, promoting the least restrictive alternatives upholding rights and helping people to hold onto their lives during a mental health crisis and last, but by no means, least, increasing the accountability of mental health services to service users.

---

8   Despite widespread appreciation for this turn to 'recovery' as an organising characteristic of progressive services, there is a critique that cautions whether the adopted notions remain too closely associated with biomedical definitions or more radical approaches have been co-opted (see Pilgrim 2008b).

9   A dedicated website, IMROC (Implementing Recovery through Organisational Change), provides a gateway to a range of resources on recovery. Available at: www.imroc.org (accessed on 21 January 2015).

Conclusions

Although experiences of compulsion are contradictory, methodological flaws and gaps in the evidence base point to a need for more rigorous studies, including more that are undertaken from a service user perspective. It is clear that many people find this experience profoundly disempowering. The issues highlighted in this chapter are ones which IMHAs will encounter when they meet 'qualifying patients', and for which they may seek redress through advocacy. Hence, IMHAs need to be alert to the overarching themes of autonomy, participation, care and recovery, how these relate to people's experience of coercion and detention and the contribution they can make to promoting self-determination in the most challenging of circumstances.

REFLECTIVE EXERCISES

1. Think about the ways in which you might come to a better understanding of what it is like to be subject to compulsion. How might an IMHA increase their understanding of what it feels like to be detained or under a CTO?

2. Consider some of the strategies IMHAs might use to ensure their practice is rooted in what is important to qualifying patients. What would they need to do?

3. From the discussion in this chapter identify the challenges and opportunities IMHAs face advocating for people subject to compulsion. Make lists of both the challenges and opportunities. What conclusions can you draw from your lists?

4. Identify what is necessary for independent advocacy to support the recovery of qualifying patients. What are the ways in which IMHAs can be 'recovery focused'? What might get in the way of practising in this way?

Chapter 6

RESEARCH AND REVIEWS OF MENTAL HEALTH ADVOCACY

Introduction

This chapter considers evaluative research and reviews of mental health advocacy. Several systematic reviews have identified that such studies are sparse (Macadam *et al.* 2013; Newbigging *et al.* 2007; Perry 2013). Research into advocacy for people using social care services generally highlights a lack of systematic research. For instance, Macadam *et al.* (2013) observe that empirical evidence is sorely lacking especially regarding cost effectiveness. The evidence base is dominated by descriptive studies and characterised by individual stories and anecdotal accounts testifying to the merits of advocacy and there is no consistent basis for assessing the evidence of advocacy's impact (Carlsson 2014; Lawton 2009; Macadam *et al.* 2013; Stewart and MacIntyre 2013). There is also little systematic published evidence that captures the experiences of advocacy partners themselves (Carlsson 2014; Perry 2013).

The lack of evidence has been attributed to a number of reasons, including advocacy organisations having to meet conflicting political objectives (Perry 2013). However, the most consistent theme is difficulty in defining advocacy such that it may not be recognised as distinct from mentoring, peer support or befriending, or that advocacy is a part of these roles (see for example Davidson *et al.* 2012) or part of professional roles, particularly social work (Fawcett 2007). Different definitions of independent advocacy and a lack of understanding of the role also contribute to the limited evidence about its effectiveness (Stewart and MacIntyre 2013). Even when it is easier to define components of an advocacy intervention, arguably as with IMHA, there is a lack of studies that have compared outcomes across advocacy partners and people not using advocacy, the notable exception being the Australian study by Rosenman, Korten and Newman (2000). Furthermore, recent systematic reviews of advocacy (Macadam *et al.* 2013; Perry 2013) have considered different types of advocacy across different populations, making it difficult to identify what might work for whom in what circumstances. Against such a backdrop, there have been a limited number of studies specifically looking at mental health advocacy, and it is to these studies specifically that we now turn in this chapter. We have restricted this narrative review to published studies, although we are aware of a number of unpublished studies that typically review provision in their local area (see for example Coleman and Dunmur 2001; Davis 2009; Martin and Mullins 2008). We have classified the published studies into four main categories, which are not exclusive, but reflect broadly different research interests:

1. *Mapping mental health advocacy needs and/or provision.* These are typically descriptive studies that have examined issues in relation to the availability of mental health advocacy and commented on needs in relation to the style of provision.

2. *Mental health advocacy in specific settings.* These are largely focused on provision in forensic or hospital settings pre-dating implementation of IMHA.

3. *Statutory advocacy.* This refers to studies that have considered statutory IMHA or IMCA. This includes research and monitoring by the CQC.

4. *Advocacy for specific groups.* This encompasses studies that have adopted a specific population focus, typically children and young people, older people or people from BAME communities. Mental health advocacy may be one aspect of wider advocacy for these groups.

Mapping studies

Many of the studies that have mapped mental health advocacy have considered needs in one place, are largely unpublished and possibly of limited value to a wider audience, although they are critically important in informing the commissioning of advocacy services at a local level. The most comprehensive published study of this kind was undertaken by Foley and Platzer (2007) who focused on services across London to identify whether provision was meeting need. Demographic data was used to estimate need and service mapping undertaken, augmented by interviews with service providers, commissioners and service users and analysis using cartographic mapping of service locations and catchment areas. The results indicated that there was reasonably equitable provision across London with each borough being served by at least one advocacy service as well as by London-wide specialist schemes. However, there were gaps in relation to the full range of specialist provision and a mismatch between need and location of specialist services, particularly for BAME groups. It was also reported that minority groups in general benefited from a style of advocacy that incorporated personal advocacy with support and working with communities, as well as instructed advocacy. This was echoed in the findings of Rai-Atkins *et al.* (2002) in their mapping of mental health advocacy in Yorkshire and the East Midlands and the extent to which this catered for African, Caribbean and South Asian communities. Overall, services were underdeveloped and mainstream advocacy services were often inaccessible to the specific needs of people from BAME communities, as discussed in more detail below.

An earlier study by Barker, Newbigging and Peck (1997) identified a sample of ten successfully established advocacy projects, as defined by either national recognition or local commendation, to identify common features of successful schemes. Interviews were undertaken with the project chair and staff, with most people interviewed being service users. The focus for these interviews was the nature of the project's development:

the current organisational arrangements for delivery and the project's own views on how it had achieved success. Of note was the limited nature of the projects, with their scope limited to people aged 25–65 years. The study provides an early indication that demand for individual advocacy, highly valued by service users, could squeeze out more strategic collective approaches. The researchers distinguished between independently established organisations rooted in user membership and 'professional' individual advocacy projects, located within a wider voluntary agency, noting that collective self-advocacy and user involvement were important features of the former but not the latter (Barker *et al.* 1997).

Advocacy in specific mental health settings

Some of the research into mental health advocacy has looked at independent advocacy on mental health wards before the introduction of IMHA in England and Wales (e.g. Carver and Morrison 2005). Other studies have focused on the experience of specific populations including patients in forensic or secure settings and involuntary patients in an Australian hospital (Barnes and Tate 2000; McKeown, Bingley and Denoual 2002; Palmer *et al.* 2012; Rosenman *et al.* 2000). There is a gap in relation to studies of advocacy support to people in community settings. One recent Scottish study (Carlsson 2014) examined the impact of IMHA provided to a broader population than those subject to compulsion, reflecting differences between English and Scottish law. Such studies have tended to be exploratory in nature, and mainly involve small samples of patients and/or staff and advocates, with the exception of Barnes and Tate (2001) and Rosenman *et al.* (2000) in Australia. Table 6.1 summarises the methods and samples used in these studies.

TABLE 6.1 SUMMARY OF THE NATURE AND SCOPE OF STUDIES IN SPECIFIC MENTAL HEALTH SETTINGS

Study details	Summary description	Methods	Sample
Barnes and Tate (2000) *Advocacy from the Outside Inside: A Review of the Patients' Advocacy Service at Ashworth Hospital.*	Review of the work and impact of the Patient's Advocacy Service at Ashworth High Secure Hospital.	Process and impact evaluation: interviews, analysis of records and literature review.	120 patients, staff, advocates and relatives.
Carlsson (2014) *Advocacy Changed My Life.*	Study of the impact of independent advocacy in the lives of people experiencing mental illness in Scotland including in-patient and community settings.	Qualitative interviews.	12 advocacy partners.
Carver and Morrison (2005) *Advocacy in practice: the experiences of independent advocates on UK mental health wards.*	Study exploring the experiences of independent advocates working with people on acute and continuing care wards.	Small-scale exploratory qualitative study of practising advocates' experiences of their work.	Convenience sample of 10 advocates.
Lacey and Thomas (2001) *A survey of psychiatrists' and nurses' views of mental health advocacy*	To examine understanding and attitudes of medical and nursing staff towards advocacy in hospital and community settings	Structured interviews	5 Senior house officers, 5 staff nurses, 4 community psychiatric nurses (CPNs) and 1 advocate

cont.

Study details	Summary description	Methods	Sample
McKeown et al. (2002) *A Review of Advocacy Services at the Edenfield Regional Secure Unit and Bowness High Dependency Unit, Prestwich Hospital.*	Study of the nature and scope of advocacy provision within secure units.	Mixed methods involving analysis of records and other documents, alongside qualitative interviews.	51 staff and patients.
Palmer et al. (2012) *Getting to know you: reflections on a specialist independent mental health advocacy service for Bexley and Bromley residents in forensic settings.*	Study of the advocacy experiences of long-term in-patients in London-based specialist forensic settings and challenging behaviour units.	Qualitative interviews.	10 service users.
Rosenman et al. (2000) *Efficacy of continuing advocacy in involuntary treatment.*	Study of individual or personal advocacy model used with detained patients in an Australian hospital setting.	Experimental design.	105 detained patients: 53 patients received personal advocacy, 52 had routine rights advocacy.

This research highlights several benefits of independent advocacy, including that it has improved the relationship between service users and professionals. Palmer *et al.*'s (2012) audit of forensic patients' experience of advocacy concluded there are 'significant gains' for service users in these settings when advocacy is introduced, and further, that there is a positive impact on service users' well-being and engagement with services. A felt need for advocacy was expressed by service users in McKeown *et al.*'s (2002) study in medium and high dependency units. The earlier Rosenman *et al.* (2000) study exploring the effectiveness of experimental personal advocacy for detained patients (i.e. an advocate assigned throughout their stay as an in-patient), compared with 'routine' advocacy (i.e. an advocate to support the patient at the early Tribunal hearing only), found higher satisfaction with treatment among those receiving personal advocacy. Other findings included lower risk of being re-hospitalised, and staff reporting advocacy as facilitating the management of patients. Carlsson's (2014) work in Scotland found that independent advocacy is a 'much needed support' for mental health service users, essential to ensuring people's rights and tackling inequality and discrimination.

In Chapter 9, exploring the values, knowledge and skills needed by IMHAs, we argue, as do Palmer *et al.* (2012), that it is essential for advocates to develop a trusting relationship with service users. Only then is advocacy a 'crucial adjunct to therapeutic and other interventions' (Palmer *et al.* 2012, p.11). These researchers also found that the preference of service users was for advocates with knowledge and understanding of the mental health system and legislation, who were able to help them navigate what can seem a complex territory, and that this was more important than matching them with an advocate of the same ethnicity or gender. This finding resonates with the results from our study and a previous study (Newbigging *et al.* 2007), which suggests that the factors involved in successful advocacy partnerships requires further exploration to better understand how to address issues of inequity.

Some of the research highlights challenges for advocates in raising concerns about poor practice at a macro level and thus making a real difference to care and treatment on wards (Carver and Morrison 2005). As we discuss in more detail in Chapter 11, the importance of developing constructive relationships between mental health staff and advocacy services, and by implication between services and service users, is strongly underlined. Staff having an appreciation of the value of advocacy and an understanding of the place of independent advocacy is identified as critical to the effectiveness of advocacy, particularly in in-patient and forensic settings. While some staff in McKeown *et al.*'s (2002) study viewed advocates as strong allies and as contributing to better treatment outcomes, some felt their professionalism was threatened by advocates and found it difficult to separate out their own role as the patient's advocate from that of an independent advocate. Furthermore, the staff in Lacey and Thomas' (2001) study, whilst appreciating the role of advocates highlighted a concern that they might promote an 'anti-medical, political agenda'.

Carver and Morrison (2005) highlight the need for training on advocacy for mental health service staff in order to tackle the inconsistent understanding of the role of advocacy, and the treatment of advocates in both acute and forensic mental health settings. Advocates in this study reported experiencing defensiveness or even hostility from clinical staff, which the researchers suggested flows in part from a lack of understanding and appreciation of the role of advocacy. Another issue was the perception of mental health staff that they are the patient's advocate, which was later highlighted as a barrier in some hospital settings by our study.

Evaluating statutory advocacy

In England and Wales, provision of independent advocacy to mental health service users as a duty under legislation only came into being under the MC Act 2005 and the MH Act 2007. Given their relative infancy therefore, it is not surprising that there are only a small number of studies that have focused on the operation and effectiveness of IMCA (Redley *et al.* 2006; Townsley and Laing 2011) and the provision of IMHA (McKeown *et al.* 2013; Newbigging *et al.* 2012a, 2014; Palmer *et al.* 2012). Most are national studies using mixed methods, except Palmer *et al.* (2012), which examined implementation of IMHA in one forensic hospital setting. Other studies relating to rights to advocacy under the law include evaluation of the early implementation of the Mental Health (Care and Treatment) (Scotland) Act 2003 (Ridley and Hunter 2013).

The relatively small body of work monitoring and evaluating the IMCA services (e.g. Banks and Redley 2009; Redley *et al.* 2006, 2009 has been characterised by a focus on process. Prior to implementation of the IMCA role under the MC Act, Redley *et al.* (2006) examined piloting the role in seven sites to provide guidance to LA commissioners. This study identified a lack of awareness of the new legislation by health and social care practitioners, as well as a number of operational dilemmas for organisations providing IMCA services. Consequently, the pilot IMCA services were found to spend a substantial amount of time raising awareness of IMCA and the MC Act, and the researchers highlighted the need for further such efforts amidst promotion of statutory advocacy, and the importance of setting up future systems to monitor service quality (Banks and Redley 2009). While there had been some improvement by the time of Townsley and Laing's (2011) study of the difference IMCAs make, they found that IMCAs were still having to act as educators and disseminators about IMCA and the MC Act with health and social care professionals.

Involvement of IMCAs had improved the clinical decision-making process by keeping service users' interests at the heart of the process, ensuring an holistic, person-centred approach was taken (Redley *et al.* 2006; Townsley and Laing 2011). In the later study of IMCA services (Townsley and Laing 2011), IMCAs reported making a significant difference to both the level of involvement in decision making for clients who were seen to lack capacity, and to the outcomes achieved for individuals. Decisions were said to be based on a more thorough assessment of the options, and IMCAs made a difference to the knowledge and practice of other professionals.

During the pilot IMCA study, a high number of ineligible referrals was made, which Redley *et al.* (2006) suggest was indicative of a gap in the provision of generic advocacy services. The researchers recommended investment in good generic advocacy as a necessity to avoid unnecessary strain on specialist IMCA resources. A later study of new mental health law in Scotland (Ridley and Hunter 2013) suggested that the demand for advocates to support service users with the Mental Health Tribunals was creating a two-tier advocacy service which privileged those subject to the Mental Health (Care and Treatment) (Scotland) Act 2003. This conclusion had also been reached by earlier commentators (Atkinson *et al.* 2007; Rushmer and Hallam 2004).

Prior to the MH Act 2007, a study carried out by Barnes, Brandon and Webb (2002), using the Delphi method to arrive at a consensus proposal, identified the need for a model of independent specialist advocacy that was: individual (i.e. one-to-one) advocacy only; to be clearly focused on those subject to the MH Act; and needing 'to operate within a spectrum of advocacy provided in a locality to meet a broad range of needs' (p.21). The model proposed has underpinned the introduction of statutory IMHA services under the MH Act 2007. Also, anticipating the introduction of IMHA services, Mind consulted with more than 150 service users, from a range of backgrounds, on what they saw as essential to the provision of successful advocacy (Mind 2006). The purpose of this was to develop standards for advocacy providers to inform both the practice and commissioning of IMHA. The framework of standards reinforced the importance of services being independent, having a service user focus and being accessible to all at times of need. Advocates' qualities were also emphasised, similar to those identified from more recent studies, i.e. excellent communication skills, empathy, creativity, reliability and trustworthiness. The consultation also highlighted the stressful nature of being sectioned and how access to an advocate can be impeded under such circumstances by lack of awareness of advocacy, lack of familiarity with the available advocate or level of personal distress. Mind recommend a range of potential solutions to promote access at a time of need including an advocacy presence on the ward, a 'soft' approach by the advocate on first meeting and the role of nursing staff in promoting access.

A year after the introduction of IMHA services, Mind sent a Freedom of Information request (FOI) to all Primary Care Trusts (PCTs)[1] in England and surveyed advocacy organisations providing IMHA services to investigate how well IMHA services were being commissioned (Hakim and Pollard 2011). The FOI requests indicated that 78 per cent of the PCTs had not put the services out to tender because of the challenging timescale for implementation. However, 'business as usual' disadvantaged particular groups as those PCTs that had not gone out to tender were less likely to have conducted a systematic needs assessment for IMHA services. Hakim and Pollard (2011) concluded that this particularly disadvantaged BAME organisations and also noted that, although IMHA services were unaware that they were not fully catering for BAME communities, they were relatively comfortable with this position. Similar to the experience with the introduction of IMCA services, levels of understanding about the IMHA role and confusion about their relationship with existing advocacy services meant that more than 80 per cent of advocacy services had received inappropriate referrals (Hakim and Pollard 2011, p.4) as well as seeing an increase.

In 2010, the Department of Health commissioned our group to undertake the first comprehensive evaluation of the quality of IMHA services (Newbigging et al. 2012a, 2014). We used a two-stage design using quantitative and qualitative methods to gather data and involved 289 stakeholders, as illustrated in Figure 6.1, to understand the experiences of IMHA and investigate the factors that influence this.

---

1   Bodies responsible for commissioning primary, community and secondary health services from 2011 to 2013. This role was assumed by Clinical Commissioning Groups on 1 April 2013.

Stage 1 What do quality IMHA services look like?	• Focused literature review of the research • 11 focus groups across England (75 participants) • Shadowing IMHAs at work • Expert panel to review and refine quality indicators

Stage 2
What is the experience of IMHA services?
What factors influence their quality and outcomes?
	• Comparative case studies of 7 NHS Trusts and 1 independent sector provider using the following methods for data collection
	  – Questionnaire to IMHA services
	  – Interviews with 214 stakeholders, including 90 'qualifying patients'
	  – Documentary analysis of key reports
	  – Analysis of IMHA service records and reports
	  – Analysis of mental health service records for evidence of impact

Figure 6.1 Overview of the design and methods for our study

Our findings indicate that the IMHA role is highly valued and appreciated by service users, although its potential was not fully realised. While aspects of the findings have been discussed throughout this book, here we highlight the three key factors that we found influence access and the quality of IMHA services: first, effective commissioning so that services meet the diversity of need and potential demand; second, supportive mental health contexts that foster constructive relationships between mental health services and advocacy services and ultimately with service users; and third, competent advocates and well-resourced advocacy services.

Our study showed that IMHA has a role to play in improving the experience and outcomes of service users under the MH Act, even if these are not always well documented (see Chapter 8 for a fuller discussion of outcomes). IMHA services contributed to better relations between service users and professionals, and to an organisational approach becoming more recovery focused. Palmer *et al.*'s (2012) study suggests that the IMHA service approach, combining formal advocacy methods with a proactive ethos, has a positive impact on engagement. Despite identifying a range of positive benefits, however, and similar to observations made by the CQC (2014a, 2015), we found that access to IMHA services was highly variable. Our study found that less than half the number of people eligible for IMHA services were accessing them, and over two-thirds of qualifying patients interviewed who had not used IMHA did not know what it was for or confused it with complaints advocacy. Similar to research into the operation of IMCA, studies of IMHA highlight a need for efforts to be invested in awareness raising and promotion of statutory advocacy to ensure people can exercise their right to be heard. A complementary study to capture experiences of the Tribunal process involving structured interviews with 152 patients who were, or had been, detained in hospital also identified that a minority had received advocacy support with the Tribunal process (Administrative Justice and Tribunals Council and CQC 2011). They, consequently, recommended that all patients should be encouraged to access IMHA services for support with the Tribunal process.

As noted earlier, mental health services have a key role to play in facilitating access to IMHA services, and understanding of each other's roles is fundamental to effectiveness. In Chapter 11 we discuss in more detail how the attitude of mental health services towards, and appreciation of, advocacy plays a key role in determining the effectiveness of IMHA (McKeown *et al.* 2014a; Newbigging *et al.* 2012a, 2014). Even some of the most knowledgeable mental health staff remained ignorant of their duty to promote this form of statutory advocacy, leading to poor access for qualifying patients. Our study highlights the need for service users to be involved in the design and delivery of training of mental health staff to foster a better understanding of the role of independent advocacy in supporting more democratic relations between service users and mental health staff (McKeown *et al.* 2014a).

A pilot study of advocacy for people with dementia, including people requiring IMCA and/or IMHA services, raised concerns about the professionalisation of advocacy and the drive towards issue-based advocacy compromising a more personal style of advocacy. This is particularly important for people with specific needs, including those relating to dementia (Brown, Standen and Khilji 2013).

Evaluating advocacy for specific groups

The number of studies that have considered mental health advocacy for specific populations is small, although several of the studies discussed above do consider access and provision for specific groups, in particular for people from BAME communities. Those that do, identify barriers in terms of access and flag up the different style of advocacy required for specific populations (see for example, Foley and Platzer 2007; Hakim and Pollard 2011; Newbigging *et al.* 2012a). The studies that have focused on specific BAME populations highlight how the conception of advocacy in particular communities differs from the mainstream conception of independent advocacy and how this influences awareness of independent advocacy by community members, preferences for the type of service and the development of a different style of advocacy within those communities. Rai-Atkins *et al.* (2002) found that the mental health advocate role was under-developed for minority groups, reflecting a lack of resources for BAME advocacy, an imbalance of power and a lack of understanding amongst mainstream mental health advocacy services of cultural issues. Mainstream advocacy services were often inaccessible and inappropriate for the needs of BAME service users, but BAME organisations were significantly less well developed than mainstream services. Similarly, Newbigging *et al.* (2007) identified a lack of awareness about entitlement, mistrust of statutory provision, different understandings of advocacy, poor partnership working between advocacy services and BAME organisations, and attitudes of mental health services to advocacy provision as barriers to access for African and Caribbean men. As noted earlier, the role of needs assessment as part of the commissioning of advocacy services is key to ensuring that diverse needs are fully met. This is supported by the findings from our study in which we identified variability in terms of commissioning IMHA services for children and young people and that little account had been taken of the needs of specific groups and of consideration of the disproportionate rates of detention of particular BAME communities, despite this having been repeatedly indicated by the CQC. We explore this issue in more detail in Chapter 10.

Similar gaps in provision have been identified for older people with dementia, and different understandings within organisations about advocacy in general and dementia advocacy in particular (Dementia Advocacy Network 2013). There were also issues for people of BAME heritage being able to access either services equipped to meet relevant cultural issues but not dementia, or geared up to provide a dementia appropriate response but lacking competence in relation to their cultural and ethnic background (Dementia Advocacy Network 2013).

Whilst some studies have noted that demographic characteristics may be less important than relational qualities (Mind 2006; Newbigging et al. 2007), it is clear that the profile of the organisation providing advocacy services is a key factor in determining access (Newbigging et al. 2007, 2014). Furthermore, the co-location with other services designed to address discrimination and social disadvantage may bring wider benefits, which are not reflected in research that has focused on advocate characteristics. PACE, a charity promoting the mental health and emotional well-being of the lesbian, gay, bisexual and transgender (LGBT) community in London, undertook a small-scale study to evaluate its mental health advocacy service (PACE 2008). This study found that combining the dual role of mental health advocacy within an LGBT service was valued by clients, who particularly valued involvement in the service.

Given the obvious limitations of such studies and the general lack of studies that have evaluated the impact of advocacy

(Macadam *et al.* 2013), there is a clear need for further research to identify the most effective organisational arrangements for providing advocacy to diverse groups. How well mainstream advocacy providers are meeting these diverse needs warrants further investigation. Issues of identity, multiple disadvantage and discrimination in a context of compulsion will clearly impact on an individual's ability to self-advocate and for mental health services to listen. The benefits of locating advocacy services within community-specific organisations, therefore, requires further investigation and we need to ask not only whether such services are more effective through providing culturally responsive and appropriate services but also in engaging with and addressing mental illness-related stigma (Westminster Advocacy Service for Senior Residents and Dementia Advocacy Network 2009).

The roots of mainstream advocacy in a predominantly White service user movement, as discussed in Chapter 3, have privileged a particular conception of advocacy as independent and instructed. The value of interdependence with other services advancing the wider interests of diverse groups and providing services may, therefore, not be fully appreciated. Furthermore, as our study shows, the emphasis on instructed advocacy means those requiring non-instructed advocacy might miss out, particularly on wards for older people which may not have a tradition of having an advocacy presence.

Conclusions

The studies reviewed highlight several key themes. While the limited number of mapping studies provide evidence of the existence of a range of (mental health) advocacy provision up and down the country, they also point up gaps such as in provision for BAME groups, in that mainstream advocacy services are often inaccessible to such groups. Also, studies as early as the 1990s (Barker *et al.* 1997) suggested that the development of individual or personal advocacy could squeeze out collective approaches. As this approach begins to dominate the development of mental health advocacy provision, there is a danger of undermining advocacy that is rooted in collective self-advocacy and user involvement. Concerns have been raised about the professionalisation of advocacy and the drive towards advocacy that is issue based (Brown *et al.* 2013). Furthermore, development of new forms of statutory advocacy impacts on the wider provision of independent advocacy, and there is some evidence that this is already creating two-tier advocacy provision, with non-statutory advocacy the poor relation. We return in the final chapter to consider the dangers of the professionalisation of advocacy in more detail.

Collectively the research reviewed in this chapter makes a convincing argument for independent advocacy provision, including in specialist settings such as forensic or secure mental health services. While, as we show in Chapter 8, there are challenges to measuring the outcomes of advocacy, the benefits of advocacy in ensuring a holistic, more person-centred approach is taken in decision-making processes have been found by several studies looking at both statutory and generic advocacy. The importance of putting the service user at the centre, and of the role of advocacy in ensuring their voice is heard, is clearly evidenced in the research findings. However, a common finding is that some professionals in health and social care have an inadequate understanding and appreciation of the role of independent advocacy, and highlighting a need for further promotion and awareness raising.

It is clear from this review that future research needs to explore the gaps in the evidence base for mental health advocacy. Of particular value would be studies that investigate advocacy outcomes and the extent to which these are influenced by contextual factors, particularly organisational models for delivery and the style of advocacy provided. This would include considering the impact of advocacy for diverse groups and the influence of different conceptions of advocacy on access and preferences for the style of advocacy. There is also a clear need for local service evaluations that consider access and uptake of different types of advocacy in specific contexts and for specific groups. In the context of compulsion, the research points to a need for studies exploring the role of advocacy in promoting empowerment of individuals as opposed to pacifying unease with coercion. There is a wider research agenda for advocacy to understand its impact on service delivery and the health and social care outcomes for advocacy partners, which would be of value to policy makers, advocacy services and people using health and social care services alike (Beaupert 2009; Macadam *et al.* 2013; Newbigging *et al.* 2014).

The way in which research is conducted has a bearing on the type of knowledge generated (Russo and Wallcraft 2011), and the majority of studies discussed in this chapter were undertaken by academic researchers. Notable exceptions are studies in which authors of this current publication were involved and, reflecting our commitment to participatory and emancipatory practices, research teams have consisted of alliances between mental health service users and academic researchers. Reflections on this experience illuminate the struggles to share power in the research process and to generate knowledge that reflects the different epistemes and experiences of service users, from diverse backgrounds, and academics (see for example, Newbigging *et al.* 2012b; Russo 2014; Russo and Wallcraft 2011).

Different modes of evaluation are also needed. Alongside summative evaluations, the value of formative methods – action research and appreciative approaches – can extend beyond the research endeavour to support local development and change the dynamic between service users, advocates and mental health professionals. There is also considerable scope for extending the role of advocates into research, both to develop their appreciation of the contribution of research and their capacity to undertake research.

REFLECTIVE EXERCISES

1. Identify (a) the benefits and (b) the challenges of IMHA highlighted by current research and evaluation.

2. Devise a future research agenda to build a better basis for assessing the value and effectiveness of independent advocacy. What would be your top three research priorities?

3. How might research priorities differ according to who draws up the research agenda? For instance, what would differ between research agendas drawn up by (a) service users/survivors; (b) advocates and advocacy services; (c) commissioners; (d) policy makers and (e) researchers? How would you go about answering these?

4. How do you think mental health service users, and/or advocates can work in alliance with academics to produce research findings that are both rigorous and relevant?

Part 2

THE PRACTICE
AND EXPERIENCE
OF INDEPENDENT
MENTAL HEALTH
ADVOCACY SERVICES

Chapter 7

THE INDEPENDENT MENTAL
HEALTH ADVOCATE
ROLE AND SERVICES

Introduction

This chapter looks at the role and responsibilities of IMHAs
and at the landscape of IMHA services across England, drawing
closely on our study as well as other recent research. In Chapter 1
we discussed different definitions and forms of (mental health)
advocacy, including self- or collective advocacy, citizen or
volunteer advocacy, and professional or paid advocacy. Here, we
focus solely on IMHA, which, as we discussed in Chapter 4 on
mental health law, is a model of statutory advocacy introduced in
2009 under the MH Act 2007. We distinguish this from IMCA,
a form of statutory advocacy implemented in 2007 under the
MC Act 2005 in England, and sometimes confused with IMHA.
Using data from our study, we sketch a unique and detailed
picture of how the IMHA service is operating, and reflect upon
its quality and effectiveness. This is supplemented by analysis of
data from a Freedom of Information request to 152 English local
authority social services departments, which highlights changes
in the service landscape since the responsibility shifted to local
authorities under the Health and Social Care Act 2012.

While local authorities have longstanding experience of
commissioning other models of advocacy for both children and
adults (e.g. generic advocacy, advocacy for children in care, self-
advocacy), the shift of responsibility for commissioning IMHA
from the NHS to local authorities, as of April 2013, represents
a substantially more radical separation of commissioning body
from mental health service providers. Subsequently, the contours

of the IMHA service landscape have been altered, driven in part by local authorities' desire to streamline processes and achieve cost effectiveness in an age of austerity, which we discuss in more detail in Chapter 12. We reflect on what these findings might mean for raising awareness of IMHA amongst all those eligible (i.e. qualifying patients), and ultimately to increasing the uptake of IMHA so that people exercise their right to be heard.

Experience of the IMHA role

There was consensus amongst advocates in our study that the legislative requirements of the IMHA role had served to raise the profile of mental health advocacy significantly and, to some extent, had broadened understandings of advocacy within mental health services. Ultimately this strengthened user involvement during and subsequent to detention. For example, the role encouraged a clear expectation of advocates' involvement in key meetings, whereas this was less so in the past. Some aspects of the statutory role, however, such as being able to speak to staff without the person being present and accessing patients' notes, were felt by some IMHAs in our study to threaten the fundamental underpinning values of advocacy that emphasise full involvement and participation of advocacy partners. They also identified tension between acting to empower and safeguard individuals' rights and being person centred. Some IMHAs we spoke to felt bounded or 'fettered' by the role as defined in the legislation and guidance. Advocates can therefore be somewhat divided in their opinions about the IMHA role, some emphasising the key importance of a boundaried role while others perceive little difference with how they previously practised (mental health) advocacy:

> Because the role is a statutory one, it's got boundaries, we've got these aims of you know helping people to understand their rights and the legislation they're being held under which is…a big change from generic advocacy where you don't have that kind of rights emphasis quite so much. (IMHA quoted in Newbigging *et al.* 2012a, p.134)

There can be differences of opinion amongst advocates about the flexibility that exists within the role and the extent to which this limits its effectiveness in meeting people's needs. In particular, in our study there were differences about the extent to which an IMHA could become involved in issues that were broader concerns for the individual than his/her rights in relation to the MH Act. IMHAs may signpost to other forms of advocacy support when previously they would have continued providing that support. Further, the boundaried focus of the role means that as soon as an individual no longer qualifies for IMHA services (i.e. they are no longer detained under the MH Act or subject to a CTO), often at the point of discharge, they may be denied access to advocacy unless the advocacy service responsible for IMHA have a strategy for ensuring continuity of access. This seems to advocates to be at odds with the foundational principles of advocacy, i.e. to be user centred, and ultimately for the individual to self-advocate, which may or may not have been achieved by the time they no longer qualify for IMHA services.

In advocacy services where the IMHA role is viewed more as a function and advocates also have the capacity to act as generic mental health advocates and/or IMCAs, there is arguably less conflict around the limitations of the IMHA role. Additionally, in our study some were of the opinion that access to IMHA should be widened from its current criteria to include voluntary or informal patients as has been done in Wales (Welsh Government 2011), and that this would go some way to reducing any role conflict:

> Why should we differentiate between informal and formal because somebody who is informal could quite easily actually meet the criteria for being sectioned and so just the fact that they've gone in as an informal patient means they're not entitled to an IMHA and I think everybody should. (IMHA quoted in Newbigging *et al.* 2012a, p.134)

IMHA services are not meant to replace other types of advocacy and support and should seek to work in conjunction with these.

Indeed, as we go on to discuss, many advocacy services offer a range of types of advocacy, with some advocates qualified to offer different advocacy roles. Nor should having an IMHA affect the individual's rights to seek legal advice. On the other hand, patients have the right to choose not to use an advocate. Our study, however, found that far from making an informed choice not to use an advocate, those patients who did not have an IMHA tended to know little about its purpose or their right to have one. Of the 29 qualifying patients we interviewed who did not have an IMHA, 67 per cent were unaware of IMHA services or were unsure if they had accessed the service because of confusion over what it is. Lack of awareness of the service was the main reason service users gave for not using IMHA. Further, several also thought independent advocacy might be a good thing and were able to identify issues that an advocate might help them with. Consequently, we recommended that 'qualifying' patients should opt out rather than have to opt into IMHA, obviating reliance on mental health staff's judgment of need to access IMHA.

Under IMHA regulations, an advocate can only act as an IMHA when specifically employed by an advocacy organisation commissioned to provide IMHA services and they must have appropriate experience and training. National guidance includes an expectation that IMHAs will normally have completed the IMHA module of the national independent advocacy qualification by the end of the first year of their practice (see Chapter 9 on doing advocacy well for more details). Our study found that, in practice, the majority of IMHAs had completed the mandatory training within 12 months of appointment. There was, however, wide variation between advocacy services, with all advocates in some services having completed the training compared to only a quarter of IMHAs in others. The vast majority of IMHAs were experienced and qualified advocates who had worked in mental health settings for a number of years, some in social work, law and other professional backgrounds.

Non-instructed advocacy

As touched upon in Chapter 4, IMHAs can work in an instructed or non-instructed way with qualifying patients. Non-instructed advocacy is where an advocate works with an individual who is unable to express his/her wishes clearly because they lack mental capacity. In such circumstances, the IMHA will represent the patient's wishes (as much as they are known) and ensure that his or her rights are respected. Indeed, some individuals may have recourse to both IMHA and IMCA. In those instances where a person qualifies for both types of statutory advocacy, the role of the IMCA is in line with the statutory guidance and will involve, for example, decisions related to medical conditions (i.e. those not covered by the MH Act). Box 7.1 provides an illustration of non-instructed advocacy and how the IMHA role extends beyond detention under the Act to address potential contributory factors.

BOX 7.1 PRACTICE EXAMPLE OF NON-INSTRUCTED ADVOCACY

The IMHA attended the advocacy partner's meetings on a non-instructed basis and was involved in the discussions concerning the partner's accommodation when his Section 2 ended. The advocacy partner's behaviour and mental health had improved after changes made to his medication and a routine had been established on the ward. During these meetings the provider of the accommodation where the partner lived expressed concerns that on discharge his behaviour would revert to how it had been before admission.

The IMHA asked the providers about the routine the partner had at home and it emerged that the partner had been banned from the communal areas and as a result spent most of his time in his room alone. The layout of the building did not allow for the partner to have anywhere else to go. The advocacy partner no longer went to day services and therefore spent all day doing nothing with very little interaction with other people. The IMHA pointed out that anyone who sat around all day alone would experience the emotions and problems that the partner had. The IMHA stated that if the routine and layout of the building did not suit the partner then it obviously was not an appropriate placement for him, and that the meeting should consider alternative accommodation where the partner would have more interaction, stimulation and activities.

The IMHA felt that there was an unenthusiastic response from the advocacy partner's supporting team, but with further input from the IMHA and the ward team another placement was found, funding agreed and the partner moved to another place of residence which was a lot busier, with outings and activities which the partner could choose to participate in or not. The partner's behaviour has since massively improved and he is keen to get involved with all that is going on. He appears to be much happier and this is reflected in his behaviour.

(Source: Provided by Cumbria County Council in response to a FOI request)

IMHAs who were working in a non-instructed way, in our study, were keen to invest as much time as possible to establish capacity, and to ensure that involving an advocate was what the person wanted:

> We always, even when working with people on a non-instructed basis, we will always still try and gain their views and wishes if we can, so the first thing that we would do is still approach them and try and communicate with them and try and sort of open up that communication. If we can't then obviously we'd need to take a step back, but we always do that prior to anything else because we want to keep that person at the centre of the decision. (IMHA quoted in Newbigging *et al.* 2012a, p.146)

Some IMHAs, in our study, felt that non-instructed advocacy compromised user-centred practice: central to how IMHA providers define their services. As one IMHA who was engaged in non-instructed advocacy remarked, it felt 'quite unnatural at first', contrasting this with generic advocacy when an advocate would not be asking for staff or family opinions unless the person had asked them to. In one area, IMHAs reported categorically never providing non-instructed IMHA, almost as a matter of principle. Many IMHAs in other areas only provided non-instructed IMHA as a last resort. In short, we found that non-instructed IMHA was quite rare. Significantly, those IMHAs who felt most comfortable adopting non-instructed advocacy approaches were those with specialist training, such as IMCA training. The importance of adopting non-instructed approaches was emphasised by one IMHA, who argued that those referred for non-instructed IMHA were likely to be the most vulnerable and, therefore, most in need of an advocate: 'Historically a lot of advocacy organisations wouldn't actually do it, but in [name of organisation] there's always been the ethos that they're the people that probably needed it the most and therefore we always have' (IMHA quoted in Newbigging *et al.* 2012a, p.147).

Typically, IMHAs acting as a non-instructed advocate followed defined procedures to ensure they did not work in a 'best interests' way by default, and that they ensured the individual was as involved as possible. The following summarises good practice steps adopted by IMHAs in our research:

- Establish whether or not the person lacks capacity or is able to communicate their wishes in some way.

- Speak with ward or community-based staff to find out about what the person communicates on a day-to-day basis and to establish any preferences.

- Look at case notes relating to the particular issue and at what has happened during their stay in hospital, for instance, and if any preferences are expressed in any way.

- Observe the person in their surroundings.

- Speak to family and/or friends to gain a picture of the person's life, how they came to be detained, what their previous living situation was like, how suitable, etc.

- Feed the results of all information gathering into decision-making meetings such as the Care Programme Approach (CPA) meetings.

This is in line with Bradley's (2008) *Framework for Change* used in the national IMHA module, which categorises approaches to working in a non-instructed way in four main ways:

- **Rights based:** this begins with the premise that we all have certain fundamental human rights that can be clearly defined and explicitly measured.

- **Person centred:** this is generally based on a long-term, trusting and mutually respectful relationship between the advocate and service user, often used within the field of learning disabilities or with young people.

- **The watching brief:** this centres around eight quality of life domains which are used as the basis for a series of questions that the advocate can put to the decision maker or service provider on behalf of the service user.

- **Witness-observer:** the advocate's role in being an observer or witness to the ways in which clients live their lives is the focus for this approach and can often be used within older people's wards and associated advocacy or within the learning disability field.

Service users' experiences of IMHA

In order to ensure service users exercise their rights and that their voice is heard, IMHAs undertake a plurality of roles and are involved in a wide range of activities to differing degrees in both hospital and community settings. Further, as acknowledged earlier, this role is conducted within challenging legal and service contexts.

Providing information to ensure individuals access their rights and entitlements under the MH Act and participate as much as possible in decisions about their care and treatment lies at the heart of the IMHA role. IMHAs can give information and advice about rights specific to particular sections of the MH Act. For some service users in our research, the IMHA was the first professional to inform them of their rights: 'She explained to me I could go with a… I never knew I could go through with the Tribunal, do you understand, that was like kryptonite in my ears' (IMHA partner, acute ward, quoted in Newbigging *et al.* 2012a, p.135).

In addition to simply providing a list of available solicitors, IMHAs could use their knowledge of how individual solicitors had represented others at Tribunals to advise on which were the best. A key aspect of what IMHAs did was to make information jargon free so that it became more accessible and understandable to service users: 'They write it down, information, what the people in the interview say and write it down in a basic language so I understand, easy language to understand' (IMHA partner quoted in Newbigging *et al.* 2012a, p.136).

Advocacy partners emphasised the importance of having someone 'on my side' at meetings such as managers' hearings, ward rounds, CPA meetings and Tribunals, which they often described as daunting. The benefits of this, as illustrated in Boxes 7.2 and 7.3, included being supported to ask questions, adding authority to the IMHA partner's voice, using knowledge about the legislative and service context to probe more deeply and taking notes to act as an aide-memoire and support reflection on the process of the meeting and its final outcome.

BOX 7.2 EXPERIENCES OF THE IMHA ROLE

I had a CPA coming up and…I wanted to have the support from the advocacy. I wanted to have a presence to kind of ask questions which I thought that if she asked, might have had more...carried more weight, if you know what I mean, if she asked the questions because I've asked questions in the past and they tend to kind of answer a question with a question. So I thought if I had the advocacy present maybe I'd get a straight answer, and she asked the questions and she done a good job and we got answers to certain questions, and it went well because not too long after that I got my leave, so I think it went well really.

(IMHA partner, medium secure unit, quoted in Newbigging et al. 2012a, p.138)

We had a young Chinese boy who had a bit of a language difficulty and some learning disability and he'd written everything down on paper that he wanted to say and the advocate actually read that out for him, which I thought was really good: a really good idea because people can gather their thoughts maybe a week or so beforehand, put it down on paper because they could find going into a room with a number of people there quite intimidating.

(MH Act administrator quoted in Newbigging et al. 2012a, p.139)

Advocacy partners tended to emphasise the IMHA's role in ensuring they were aware of, and were able to exercise, their rights, including the right to appeal through the Tribunal system. From the service user perspective, therefore, IMHAs play an invaluable role in ensuring the user voice is heard in the system. However, our study found stark differences between areas in the involvement of IMHAs at Tribunals despite official recognition for their role supported by guidance issued in 2011 (Ministry of Justice 2011). IMHAs reported Panel members' and the Chair's uncertainty about their role at Tribunals: 'It depends very much on the Tribunal or the Chair and who's managing the Tribunal. Some are more kind of engaging and some of them you know, "what are you doing here?" really' (IMHA quoted in Newbigging *et al.* 2012a, p.139). This uncertainty was echoed by some advocacy partners: 'I don't think there's much point an advocate attending my Tribunal because they [Panel] only really listen to the lawyers really' (Newbigging *et al.* 2012a, p.139).

Across the sample in our study, IMHAs were variously described in active roles of 'god motherly person', a 'lever' or a 'hammer', essentially because they had made something happen. Other service users described the IMHA role as more of a negotiator within the system, using words such as 'diplomat' or 'bridge' about the IMHA, or that they were the 'WD40' in the system, although this could mean either that they helped move things on for the service user or, more negatively, that they simply maintained the status quo: 'That's why I've described her as WD40…it's been necessary for me to have her to almost smooth over some of these disjointed problems that occur from me being shoved around' (IMHA partner quoted in Newbigging *et al.* 2012a, p.133). For another person, the IMHA acted as a 'witness' to the poor treatment she had experienced in the mental health service system, and similarly, other advocacy partners referred to a safeguarding role performed by IMHAs:

> It's nice to have somebody like N or one of her associates to be there as a witness to it all and see what they get up to, and put a stop to certain events that they could get up to. (IMHA partner on a CTO quoted in Newbigging *et al.* 2012a, p.133)

Although the prime purpose of advocacy is to support people to have a voice, IMHAs bring an understanding of the legislative and service context to this task, as illustrated in Box 7.3.

BOX 7.3 PRACTICE EXAMPLE OF IMHA SUPPORT AT A HOSPITAL MANAGER'S MEETING

The advocacy partner had seven hours' Section 17 leave every day and was using this time appropriately to go home to her flat – always returning to the ward at the agreed time with no issues. The IMHA went through the hearing reports with the partner to clarify any points and give her an opportunity to comment and explain her view. The reports seemed to be very negative on the questions about risks in the community and steps that could be taken to support her if she were discharged. The IMHA was unsure of the reason for a continued section as there were no problems with returning from leave or with accepting medication. It seemed that the only reason for detention was lack of accommodation as the provider of the flat the partner currently lived in had stated they were unable to house her any longer as they could not manage her behaviour effectively. The IMHA also noticed that the partner had previously been under section in November of last year and funding had been applied for to provide a care package. It had also been planned for the partner to be placed on to a CTO which she had agreed to. Unfortunately funding for the full package had not been agreed and the Responsible Clinician decided she did not require a CTO, the advocacy partner was discharged and didn't have full support in place.

At the hearing the IMHA raised these issues and suggested that the partner had not been supported appropriately, which may have led to the current admission. This was supported further by the chairperson of the meeting who had been involved with the partner on her previous admission, even attending her multi-disciplinary team (MDT) meetings on the ward to ensure the right package was in place. He was extremely disappointed the full care package had not been agreed and that he had not been informed of this as he had asked to be at the time.

As a result of the hearing it was agreed that a repeat bid for the complete funding would be made with the support of the Hospital Managers. The provider agreed to accept the advocacy partner back to the flat on this basis – the extra funding would enable them to employ night staff to support her, which was raised as a still cheaper option than funding a placement out of county.

The Managers upheld the section with a review booked in four weeks – after the funding decision had been made by the commissioners. It was also agreed that the chairperson of the Hospital Manager's panel would attend all ward rounds for the partner until discharge.

(Source: Provided by Cumbria County Council in response to a FOI request)

Rarely had IMHAs in our study accessed patient records. It was invariably the case that mental health service staff were unaware of the right of IMHAs to access patient records. Given this was only an occasional occurrence, it tended to be considered a non-issue. Accessing patients' notes posed a dilemma for some advocates:

> I've avoided that, looking at the records because of the clause that we can't share everything. If there is something we can't share with the service user…and as a passionate advocate I suppose I wouldn't ever want to be in that position. (IMHA quoted in Newbigging *et al.* 2012a, p.144)

In some areas there were clear protocols between the NHS Trusts and advocacy services, including controlled access to NHS databases, facilitating access. Where this right had been exercised, it had been a valuable check of whether and how opinions had been recorded, and what follow-on actions had been formalised – for example:

> What I was aiming to do, and well he said to me, 'I've filled in the form asking them to find me a solicitor.' So I said, 'Is it okay with you if I ask the staff that allows me to see that?' And he said, 'Yeah of course it is.' So I then went to the member of staff, saw the record, I saw it for myself, nobody had done anything about it. Shocking. Because that's a person's life. (IMHA quoted in Newbigging *et al.* 2012a, p.145)

IMHA provision: a variable landscape

Research undertaken in 2011 by Mind (Hakim and Pollard 2011), together with our research study, indicated that provision of IMHA across England tended to be uneven, and the organisations providing IMHA varied significantly from national providers, such as Rethink, Mind or the CAB, to small local or regional advocacy services. A mapping study of mental health advocacy services in London in 2006 (Foley and Platzer 2007) similarly found provision to be patchy with no single borough having the full range of specialist provision to match local need. Our study found that the number of advocacy services providing IMHA to different hospital populations can vary greatly, with some having just one advocacy provider to relate to while others have seven or more different IMHA providers. Not only can there be multiple advocacy services, in some areas there can be multiple health bodies to relate to: for example, in two areas, five different advocacy services provided IMHA across seven PCTs, and in another, four different IMHA providers were commissioned by five PCTs. The potential for confusion about which agencies are providing IMHA in these circumstances was great.

The change in commissioning responsibility for IMHA services moving to local authorities has changed this landscape further. The number and range of advocacy services providing IMHA has been rationalised as local authorities have sought to encourage 'one stop shops' for advocacy from organisations offering the full range of advocacy support. This clearly favours larger advocacy providers over small local organisations. In one of the eight areas in our study there were four different advocacy services providing IMHA to the NHS target population, which had been rationalised to one by 2013 plus another servicing secure provision. A response to the FOI request, responded to by 103 local authorities in England, showed 86 per cent commissioning just one IMHA provider, while 10 per cent commissioned the service from two different providers. Only 2 per cent reported having three or more IMHA providers, and 2 per cent had commissioned local consortiums consisting of multiple advocacy organisations working in a partnership arrangement.

Similar to earlier research (Hakim and Pollard 2011), our earlier study found that the majority of IMHA providers were well-established advocacy organisations, operating since the mid- to late 1990s, with a minority having been in existence for over 30 years. Many PCTs had continued to contract with existing advocacy providers when IMHA was implemented in 2009 (Hakim and Pollard 2011). This picture was confirmed by our study, finding that just a third of providers were relatively new organisations, and only two had been set up in 2009 specifically to provide IMHA. In other words, most were experienced advocacy providers providing support (though not statutory advocacy) to people under the Mental Health Act 1983, and had been subsequently commissioned to provide IMHA from 2009 on the 'basis of our reputation' or because of 'having skilled advocates'.

The FOI results show the greatest proportion of advocacy organisations commissioned in 2014 by local authorities and CCGs to provide IMHA were national organisations, followed by regional and local advocacy organisations (see Figure 7.1). National organisations included Rethink and Voiceability, while regional organisations included Mind. The type of organisation being commissioned at a local level was, arguably, more reflective of a rights-based focus. For example, this included organisations that were part of a broader coalition around rights in relation to disabled people's rights, or general rights through co-location with Citizens' Advice, or were situated with organisations that provided a broad range of services including housing and welfare rights for people with mental health issues.

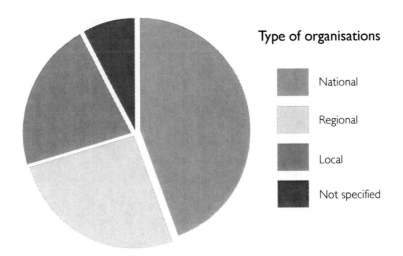

Figure 7.1 Type of organisations being commissioned
to provide IMHA services by local authorities

The research findings therefore indicate that the interface between mental health services and advocacy services can be very complex; our study found that some hospitals and community mental health services were relating to multiple IMHA providers covering diverse populations, while others had just one provider. The latter was particularly the case for secure hospital populations. As noted above, this situation has changed since the shift of commissioning. In our study, conducted between 2010 and 2012, we found some confusion about who provided IMHA and a lack of awareness of local IMHA provision amongst mental health service staff, especially when the hospital had a wide catchment area and there were multiple IMHA providers to relate to.

As Table 7.1 demonstrates, there can be wide variation in understanding and awareness of both the IMHA role and the providers of IMHA. We also found confusion with IMCA, with IMHA and IMCA being used synonymously and interchangeably by mental health service staff. Mental health service staff working in Community Mental Health Teams (CMHTs) and supporting those on CTOs were the most likely to confuse these two forms of statutory advocacy. Taken together with findings that showed that as few as a fifth of qualifying patients were accessing IMHA in some areas, this would suggest that staff's awareness directly impacts on uptake.

TABLE 7.1 MENTAL HEALTH SERVICES STAFF'S AWARENESS OF IMHA			
Percentage of staff asked who were able to recall name of IMHA or of the service	Percentage of staff who showed confusion with IMCA	Percentage of staff interviewed who understood it was their duty to inform qualifying patients about IMHA	Percentage of staff interviewed that knew IMHAs can access records
15–100, influenced by organisational changes.	18–45, but community mental health staff had little contact.	20–86 understand it is an obligation.	10–30.

The existence of multiple IMHA providers was perceived by advocates and mental health services staff as problematic, as it led to confusion about which organisation to contact about IMHA for particular patients. Commissioning practices and the differential development of advocacy in local areas will impact on how IMHA is provided. Given that the FOI request (2014) found a majority of local authorities had commissioned one IMHA provider, this may be changing for the better. However, as local authority boundaries are not necessarily co-terminus with those of mental health trusts, this may still be an issue for mental health staff.

Spectrum of advocacy services

The model of independent specialist advocacy proposed by Barnes *et al.* (2002), which underpinned the introduction of IMHA, operated within a spectrum of advocacy so that a broad range of needs could be met. Unsurprisingly, we found only a minority of advocacy services specialised in IMHA alone. Our FOI request (2014) also found that just a quarter of local authorities commissioned IMHA only, with the majority commissioning a mix of advocacy support including IMHA, IMCA, DOLS, generic mental health advocacy and complaints advocacy. It is likely that such commissioning practices will further encourage development of multi-model advocacy provision to meet a range of needs.

Our study found that providers tend to offer a mix of statutory IMHA and IMCA services, generic mental health, citizen or volunteer advocates, and a range of peer and self-advocacy support, meeting a variety of needs. Most commonly such agencies offered generic mental health advocacy (61%) and a few also offered IMCA (39%). Few advocates were trained as both IMHA and IMCA. In services where they were, it was the stated vision to have 'highly trained advocates' who could operate in both capacities, whereas other services considered them separate specialisms. One explanation for the separation may lie in the different funding and commissioning mechanisms operating at the time of the research, which has since changed. Providing generic mental health advocacy as well as IMHA arguably enabled a more holistic or seamless approach to meeting people's needs:

> It's an advantage to the patients that I can do both because I don't then have cut off points where I say 'oh well you're voluntary now so I'm not advocating for you any more'.... If I'm doing something for somebody and they're discharged or they leave the unit, I will continue advocating for them until their issues are resolved or they're happy and satisfied. (IMHA quoted in Newbigging *et al.* 2012a, p.115)

In contrast, another IMHA who had moved from an agency providing broad-based advocacy services to one purely offering an IMHA service drew attention to the limitations of specialising in one form of advocacy: 'It's very difficult to say no to patients... You want to go in there and take on everyone's human rights and work with everybody and that's something we can't do because of the statutory obligations' (IMHA quoted in Newbigging *et al.* 2012a, p.115). Flexibility can be achieved through IMHAs operating within larger advocacy organisations that provide a range of forms of advocacy. A minority view in our study was that the same advocate adopting different roles could lead to confusion, in particular for ward staff. Although common, it was not invariably the case that IMHAs also acted as generic mental health advocates.

IMHA workforce

Our study was the first to look in detail at the characteristics of IMHA services, including exploring some aspects of the IMHA workforce. We found a predominantly female (73%) and White (84%) workforce, resonating with an earlier analysis of advocacy personnel undertaken by Action for Advocacy (2008). However, the obvious lack of choice in advocates was not raised as an issue by advocacy partners. The gender, ethnicity or disability characteristics of IMHAs proved far less important to service users than advocates' training, personal and relational qualities, and their perceived effectiveness in supporting the individual's agenda. There was also an understanding that in some services with only one advocate providing IMHA, choice of any kind was simply impracticable. It was suggested that the short-term nature of the relationship meant such choice was in fact less pressing an issue than it would be in longer-term advocacy partnerships:

> Why do I need a choice? ... If they do their job professionally then it doesn't matter whether you get on with them or not... In an emergency situation when you need someone, they just need to be professional and know their job. If at a later date you don't get on with that person then you could be offered choices. (IMHA partner quoted in Newbigging *et al.* 2012a, p.119)

Nonetheless, the nature of the IMHA workforce clearly limits opportunities for meeting individual preferences, particularly in terms of cultural and ethnic diversity, but also in terms of age and gender, as most were mature women over 40 years. In some advocacy services, all the IMHAs were female. Cases were sometimes allocated along gender lines if there was a mix of male and female IMHAs, and in some instances such allocation had been critical:

> I asked one of my male colleagues to take that case because I was uncomfortable with it and they did that and things completely changed. For safety reasons, I've had to change because it came about that there was a significant risk to females with one particular person and again I did highlight that to my manager. (IMHA quoted in Newbigging *et al.* 2012a, p.120)

Operational issues

While it is impossible to define a typical IMHA case, our study indicates that IMHAs tend generally to work with their advocacy partners for a relatively short time, with 62 per cent of IMHA providers reporting cases being open for one to three months. Advocacy services, however, varied greatly in their practice, with some averaging open cases of four to six months, and others an average of seven to twelve months. The majority (87%) reported working in an open-ended way and found it impossible to generalise, although one advocacy service specified on average four hours for IMHA involvement in CPA and six hours for Tribunal work, and another reported that they allocated each ward a minimum of two visits per week but that all advocacy partners were seen in pre-CPA meetings for six-monthly reviews. It is likely that future working practices will be influenced by demand and the resources allocated to meet this.

Findings from our study suggest that practice is not easily standardised across local areas and this can be seen in the finding that an IMHA's caseload size varies greatly. Taken across the whole sample, an IMHA was estimated to be working with

25 individuals, although some had only eight while others had 55 advocacy partners. This may also reflect the different practices within advocacy services of advocates specialising in IMHA whilst others take on wider responsibilities. Size of caseload did not appear to be associated with either the number of IMHAs in a service, the make-up of advocates' caseloads (i.e. percentage of caseload that was IMHA), or whether or not cases remained live for a fixed or open period. On average, an advocate with a mixed caseload tended to a 60:40 IMHA ratio of generic mental health advocacy cases. Advocacy managers indicated that cases tended to be allocated to IMHAs on the basis of capacity, but that some specialised in working with individuals with hearing impairment or with non-instructed advocacy. This was obviously limited by the small pool of available IMHAs within advocacy services.

Conclusions

In this chapter we have considered aspects of the experience of the IMHA role and provision of IMHA services. On one level, IMHA is a form of statutory advocacy with a clearly defined role and parameters, while on another it can be viewed as restrictive and limiting if the need for advocacy is not met once an individual stops being a qualifying patient and the advocacy service does not have capacity to offer other forms of advocacy. One area where there seems to be wide variation in practice is in the use of non-instructed approaches. Nonetheless, the importance of IMHAs working in this way cannot be underestimated; the most vulnerable people including older people with dementia and people with learning disabilities are amongst those with least access to IMHA. Whatever the viewpoint, advocates seem unanimous in the view that making mental health advocacy a statutory duty, even if only for those under compulsion, has raised the profile and importance of advocacy and that this can only be a good thing.

The research discussed in this chapter shows variability in the roles undertaken by IMHAs. While practice supports the legislative emphasis on ensuring service users understand and exercise rights and entitlements under the MH Act, supporting participation in decision making and enabling their voice to be heard, this role is directly affected by how well mental health services staff and others (e.g. Tribunal members) understand and appreciate the advocacy role. IMHA is also experienced by some service users as a significant safeguard when faced by services that disempower them and do not treat them with respect.

That mental health services staff potentially will have to relate to a multitude of advocacy providers indicates the challenges facing the promotion of IMHA to qualifying patients. Staff may well not know all of the agencies providing IMHA in their local catchment area, and it is incumbent upon advocacy services to ensure there is good promotional material. The Social Care Institute for Excellence (SCIE) and the University of Central Lancashire (UCLan) have developed a number of resources in co-production with service users to promote understanding and awareness of the right to IMHA services (see UCLan/SCIE 2015 in the Useful Resources section).

The apparent rationalisation of IMHA providers across the country in the wake of the Health and Social Care Act 2012 and the shift of commissioning responsibility to local authorities may be simplifying the IMHA landscape. However, problems arising from the lack of co-terminus boundaries between health and local authorities may still continue to exacerbate this. Further, the range of advocacy providers across the country appears to have reduced in favour of larger national organisations, which may have an impact on the ability of providers to meet the specialist needs of some groups, especially those from BAME communities. Our findings, that as few as 40 per cent of qualifying patients have been able to access IMHA services, suggest that it is important to address any gaps in understanding and awareness of IMHA services amongst mental health services staff and qualifying patients.

REFLECTIVE EXERCISES

1. List some of the challenges that IMHAs face in fulfilling their role. How might IMHAs work to mitigate these challenges, for example providing non-instructed IMHA services, or accessing patients' notes?

2. Think of scenarios when it would be beneficial to an individual who is assessed as lacking capacity to have both an IMHA and IMCA and how this might work. In practice, what might the challenges be for advocates operating across this interface?

3. You are tasked with designing a seamless advocacy service that meets a range of needs, including for people under compulsory measures. What would its key features be? How could you ensure you optimised effectiveness, including cost effectiveness?

4. Think of some situations when non-instructed IMHA would be appropriate and consider how the IMHA should practise to ensure the individual is as involved as possible. What training might IMHAs need to practise non-instructed advocacy within their remit?

Chapter 8

MAKING A DIFFERENCE

The Impact of Independent Mental Health Advocacy

Introduction

This chapter explores the difference that IMHA services can make to the lives of people detained under the MH Act. The main goal of IMHA services is that an individual is able to speak for themselves as a consequence of support from an IMHA. Ideally, this is in relation to a care team that is open to hearing and involving that person in decisions about their care and treatment (Newbigging *et al.* 2014). For most stakeholders, the impact for individual service users is the most important consequence or measure of the effectiveness of any advocacy (Brandon and Brandon 2000). It is clear, however, that there are different stakeholder perspectives on what it is important to achieve, and these will influence the focus for evaluation of IMHA services locally.

There have, however, been several recent reviews that have rehearsed the challenges of identifying outcomes as a result of advocacy (Macadam *et al.* 2013; Townsley, Marriott and Ward 2009). Embedded in this difficulty are the various ways in which the impact of advocacy is framed in respect of:

1. the focus of the impact – is it for service users, staff or services?

2. the type of impact – is it empowering and transformational or does it constitute a pacification process that leaves the status quo largely intact?

3. the quality of the impact – are relevant outcomes a matter of degree, worked out differently, for different people, in different contexts?

These categories of outcome are not mutually exclusive and can be seen to relate to each other. The potential for IMHA services to make a difference is strongly affected by other themes explored throughout this book: namely, the qualities, interpersonal style and effectiveness of particular advocates and advocacy services; the adequacy of investment in those services; the extent to which host mental health services and practitioners welcome advocacy and are prepared to support its involvement; and the complexities and configurations of these settings and the attendant legal frameworks, not least compulsion into services. The task of evaluating the difference advocacy makes is clearly challenging, and this chapter aims to explore how this task might be best approached.

One common error in evaluating impact, particularly in the routine monitoring of services, is the confusion between an 'output' and 'outcome'. An output refers to the activity or participation that results in an outcome, and whilst outputs are important to understand they do not illuminate the impact for an individual. For example, an output that commissioners will be interested in is how many people the IMHA service has supported in the last year and what type of support was offered but, on its own, this tells us nothing about what difference the support given has made to the advocacy partners' lives. The ease with which output information can be captured can skew the focus away from outcomes, so it is important to have a clear understanding of the difference between them (Miller 2011).

Outcomes can be conceived of as short, medium and long term, and Miller (2011, p.2) summarises three different types of outcomes:

- **Quality of life outcomes**: the aspects of the person's whole life that they are working to achieve or maintain, and this will include relationships, housing, employment and a decent income

- **Process outcomes**: relates to the experience that people have of seeking, obtaining and using services and supports, and goes beyond satisfaction with the service

- **Change outcomes**: relates to changes in personal circumstances, including well-being, confidence, relationships and the nature of support from services.

Theory of change approaches, for example using logic modelling, provide a useful way of expressing and linking outputs, process outcomes and change outcomes (both short term and long term) and of bringing together different types of data (quantitative and qualitative) to provide a comprehensive picture of impact. Such models can provide a framework for local evaluation, and we consider a logic model for IMHA services before concluding with suggestions on methods for capturing relevant data on the impact of IMHA services.

What difference can advocacy make?

Although it may be accepted that an individual is able to speak for themselves, it is the most important consequence or measure of the effectiveness of any advocacy (Brandon and Brandon 2000), there are likely to be different stakeholder perspectives on what it is important to achieve.

As illustrated in the previous chapter, benefits of advocacy that are commonly identified include empowerment of individuals; improved quality of life; improved access to a range of care and support options; improved communication between service users and professionals; and wider improvements in services (Wetherell and Wetherell 2008). In their scoping review of the evidence of impact of advocacy in social care generally, Macadam *et al.* (2013) identify a wide range of potential impacts, as summarised in Box 8.1. Consistent with Townsley *et al.* (2009) and findings from our study, they distinguish between the benefits that arise from the process of advocacy and the outcomes that advocacy achieves (i.e. process outcomes and change outcomes) and which will contribute to an individual's overall quality of life.

BOX 8.1 PROCESS OUTCOMES AND CHANGE OUTCOMES FOR ADVOCACY

Process outcomes

These are:

- having a voice and being listened to

- increased knowledge of and ability to obtain rights and entitlements

- increased ability to make informed decisions and be involved in decision making

- ability to plan for self and keep well when supported by an advocate

- better communication and relationships between individuals and professionals, including improved communications through understanding of cultural issues for individuals from BAME communities

- feeling reassured and having someone on side, regardless of end outcomes

- increased opportunities for participation in the community, supporting people to take part in democratic processes and taking part as active citizens.

Change outcomes

These are:

- increased confidence

- increased choice and control

- increased independence

- increased feeling of being safe and secure

- improved health and well-being, including reduced mental distress

- greater empowerment and personal development

- increased access to services

- increased membership of networks and improvements in personal relationships.

(Source: Adapted from Macadam et al. 2013)

The impact of IMHA services identified from our study resonate with these, as illustrated in Table 8.1.

TABLE 8.1 SUMMARY OF IDENTIFIED IMPACTS OF IMHA IN RELATION TO PROCESS AND OUTCOMES	
Process outcomes	**Change outcomes**
Ensuring service users have a voice Increasing service users' confidence Someone alongside, on your side Providing information to increase understanding of options Feeling supported and empowered Safeguarding rights	Service users' understanding and knowledge of rights and of treatment increased Helped towards service users' recovery and increased sense of well-being Service users empowered to exercise rights Service user participation in decisions affecting their care and treatment Acceptance of the status quo Successful resolution of complaints

(Source: Newbigging et al. 2012a, p.192)

Alongside this, it can also be helpful to consider the level at which a difference is made. From conceptual mapping of data from focus groups with African Caribbean men who were service users, six key themes were identified where advocacy needs to make a difference (Newbigging *et al.* 2007):

- personal development in terms of increased confidence and ability to get on with other people and with life

- changes in the family and/or support system, including increased awareness and acceptance of mental health issues and activating more support from family, friends and communities

- changes in relationships between services and individuals so that people have greater choice and control, are more involved in care planning, can negotiate changes in treatment, particularly medication, and where there is attention to and resolution of problems resulting in better engagement and greater satisfaction with service provision

- changes in care and treatment, including improved access to services, a greater range of treatments, more quickly delivered, more consistently and to a higher standard, and diversion from restrictive forms of care including less use of in-patient services and compulsion

- changes in service provision and organisational culture so that services are more culturally appropriate and, therefore, more effective

- changes in the social and civil status of the individual, with greater independence from mental health services and increased participation in civic and social roles.

They mirror the outcomes identified by Macadam *et al.* (2013), placing advocacy in a mental health context and emphasising the importance of civic status, reflecting both the mental illness-related stigma and particulars of social disadvantage, in this instance that experienced by African and Caribbean men in relation to mental health services (Mclean, Campbell and Cornish 2003).

The way in which these outcomes overlap is illustrated in Figure 8.1, bringing together different levels at which advocacy services can make a difference.

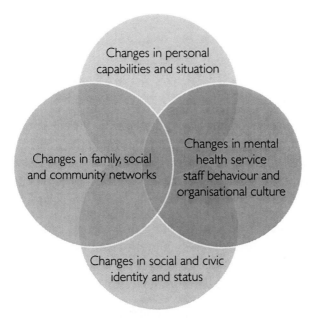

Figure 8.1 Levels at which advocacy services can make an impact (Source: Adapted from Newbigging et al. 2007)

Conceptualising the different levels at which advocacy can have an impact raises questions about the extent to which IMHA services engage with wider realities of daily living. These broader quality of life issues will clearly be harder to change than the immediate practical issues, and advocacy may not make a tangible difference to an individual's basic circumstances, such as holding onto a job or changing their accommodation (Bowes and Sim 2006; Macadam *et al.* 2013), but remains an important strand of evaluating impact if IMHA is located within a recovery-focused approach.

Service user-defined outcomes for IMHA services

The starting point for evaluating IMHA services is to identify what people subject to compulsion want those services to achieve for them. Involving service users, having a voice, getting off a section, participating in decisions affecting their care and treatment and improving the relationship with mental health staff are recurrent themes.

Having a voice

The importance of having an ally, someone alongside you to speak up for you or support you to speak for yourself, when subject to the MH Act, is clear and was highlighted in the response to experts by experience to the consultation in the revisions to the Code of Practice for the MH Act:

> You could ask almost anyone using mental health services what really matters to them and they would say the same: The one thing that makes a difference is knowing that your voice is being heard. (Department of Health 2014b, p.6)

This emphasis on voice resonates with the idea of advocacy as a mechanism for addressing epistemic injustice and crucially that their interpretations of personal experiences of distress are not discounted:

> I felt like I was being punished. I felt like I was on remand rather than in hospital, and it was nice that I had the advocate because I felt like it was the only voice I had apart from my own. (IMHA partner, psychiatric intensive care unit (PICU), quoted in Newbigging *et al.* 2012a, p.193)

Supporting service user voice has a number of intrinsic benefits, most crucially affirmation and being valued as a person reflected in enhanced self-confidence and a positive sense of agency and identity, recalibrating the balance of power in favour of the service user so that they feel less powerless. The value of feeling listened to is sometimes framed as having a therapeutic effect, promoting resilience and well-being. It is clear that there are benefits from advocacy even when involvement of an IMHA does not achieve the service user's initial goals:

> Practically there wasn't much of a difference, the doctor didn't respond to her and her suggestions but I felt more empowered, I felt more able to get the right outcomes with somebody there who was on my side. She made me feel like, yes I can deal with these issues that I wasn't getting anything, any help with. She made me feel empowered. (IMHA partner quoted in Newbigging *et al.* 2012a, p.194)

Getting off a section

As we observed in Chapter 6, research on the impact of independent (mental health) advocacy on care and treatment is sparse. However, as we found in our study, IMHA partners commonly want advocates to get them off a section and link the value of having a voice in the process as enabling them to achieve this goal. Perry (2013) concluded from a systematic review of advocacy outcomes that advocacy may significantly reduce the length of hospitalisation, reduce readmission rates, increase quality of life and increase the level of other resources used by service users. However, these conclusions are drawn from studies that were not solely focused on involuntary hospitalisation and the evidence base in this regard is underdeveloped.

The findings of our study suggest that IMHAs helped qualifying patients get off a section quicker than they might have through adopting a safeguarding role and upholding rights under the MH Act 1983. The importance of understanding your situation and having information about your rights and the compulsory measures you are subject to go some way to mitigating the sense of powerlessness and bewilderment with being compulsorily detained:

> They will tell you what they're going to do, note down everything you say, tell you what they're going to do and keep you informed on things so that you know exactly where you

are and what's going to happen. (IMHA partner, acute ward, quoted in Newbigging *et al.* 2012a, p.195)

IMHA support can go further than this to support people to exercise their rights, by helping them access a solicitor, or supporting them in hearings and Tribunals, so that they can appeal against the section. Our study found that when there is little indication that IMHAs are influencing decisions regarding sections, IMHA partners can be left feeling dissatisfied with advocacy and relatively powerless in the face of the system. This fuels scepticism about the potential of IMHA to maintain the status quo (McKeown *et al.* 2013).

Participation in decisions affecting care and treatment

As discussed in Chapter 5, the exclusion from decisions affecting care and treatment under the MH Act leaves people feeling that their autonomy has been violated. Despite the circumstances of detention, our study emphasised that people want to have a say in their treatment, to have leave to get off the ward and to make changes in medication. The experience of greater participation has wider ramifications for self-esteem:

> She [IMHA] was able to help me get some leave and that was good for me. Getting off the ward was beneficial to me and the fact that she helped me be able to kind of cheat the system a bit so that I wasn't detained under the Section 3, that helped me a lot because I'd given up. She helped me to have some time away from the hospital to start to think and to start to realise that life outside wasn't quite as awful as I perceived it to be. So she did help me get better by enabling me to have something positive happen. (IMHA partner on a CTO quoted in Newbigging *et al.* 2012a, p.199)

The research evidence suggests that advocacy has been less successful in bringing about change in levels of participation in care and treatment such as the person being able to exercise choice through a broader range of options being offered and discussed.

Improving the relationship with mental health staff

Allied to greater participation in decision making and improved choices is change in the relationship with mental health services staff, typically framed as being treated with respect by staff, reducing the adverse experiences or actions that happen, successfully resolving complaints and having a more positive experience of ward rounds or Tribunals. The sheer presence of an IMHA was identified in our study as having an impact on the behaviour of staff; by 'opening this place up the more the light comes on it and the more open and transparent it becomes' (Newbigging *et al.* 2012a, p.196). This suggests that IMHAs can have an impact on ward culture as well as on the behaviour and attitudes of individual staff. This was not only the case in hospital settings; some of those under CTOs also mentioned the importance of the advocate's safeguarding function, suggesting that the presence of an IMHA in meetings with professionals had shifted the way professionals related to and spoke to the service user.

Different perspectives on the impact of IMHA services

In our study, in contrast to service users' views, IMHAs and mental health professionals explicitly framed the impact of advocacy in terms of the legislative context, that is, protecting service users' rights in relation to the MH Act. Mental health staff identified a reduction in complaints and greater concordance with care plans as an important outcome, whilst IMHAs, echoing the view of detained patients, identified leave or discharge from a section as key. In a follow-on piece of work with a range of stakeholders, IMHAs also defined impact in terms of people being treated with greater dignity, with respect for their issues and demonstrable changes in the system. In contrast, commissioners highlighted equitable access to IMHA services as something they are interested in, although arguably this is an output rather than an outcome. They were also keen to see greater awareness and increased understanding amongst detained patients and mental health staff of rights, the legal framework and of the measures people were subject to. Underpinning this difference in priorities might be differences in the terms used to describe outcomes and advocacy – for example, 'indicators' is often used in a health context, or the term 'safeguarding vulnerable adults' is used to refer to non-instructed advocacy (Action for Advocacy 2009). This underlines the importance of local stakeholders discussing and agreeing the focus for evaluation.

The challenge of evaluating the impact of advocacy

Brandon and Brandon (2000) argue that there is a pressing need to understand the effectiveness of advocacy if it is to survive, or: 'put bluntly do advocates get what their clients are asking for?' (p.7). This is often posed as the starting point for understanding whether or not advocacy is making a difference (Action for Advocacy 2009) but, in the absence of a framework for thinking about potential impacts, may make it difficult to establish whether the impact could have been greater than was actually achieved. It is also possible, and particularly in the context of compulsion, that what some people want reflects that their assessment of the possibilities has been dulled by the circumstances in which they now find themselves.

From the above, it can be seen that there is complexity in terms of understanding the difference that IMHAs can make to the lives of people subject to compulsion. Individual advocacy projects (see Action for Advocacy 2009; Broadbridge 2012) have developed and promoted tools for capturing information on outcomes, but no single evaluation framework exists (Bauer *et al.* 2013). Consensus regarding the challenge of making sense of advocacy's impact exists in a context of scarcity of evidence, reasons for which include the following:

- Advocacy can be framed solely in terms of the quality of the relationship and the process of moving towards a goal and developing the potential of people rather than the achievement of a final state or change (Action for Advocacy 2009).

- Advocacy may be one of many influences or interventions in a person's life that bring about change, and it is therefore difficult to attribute the change to advocacy and demonstrate cause and effect (Action for Advocacy 2009; Miller 2011).

- People using advocacy services may be unable to clearly identify or express goals and/or outcomes (Action for Advocacy 2009), and this is particularly pertinent to people who are subject to compulsion and may be unclear or distressed during early meetings with an IMHA, as well as those lacking capacity to instruct an advocate.

- Advocacy aims to facilitate a change in the power of the service user, and what the individual does with the increased power is up to them, resulting in diverse and potentially contradictory success outcomes (Action for Advocacy 2009; Macadam *et al.* 2013; Perry 2013; Stewart and MacIntyre 2013).

- Defining and measuring outcomes may be viewed as being in conflict with advocacy principles, notably being person centred, non-judgmental and not imposing views or opinions (Action for Advocacy 2009).

- Responses can be influenced by service user characteristics unrelated to the quality of advocacy services, such as age, gender, region of residence, self-reported health status, type of care and expectations (Raleigh and Foot 2010).

The consequences of this are that information collated about IMHA services is either minimal or restricted to activity information or individual stories (not thematically analysed), making it difficult to make comparisons across the advocacy sector on the effectiveness of IMHA services. As well as making the case for improvements to evaluating the difference that IMHA services can make at a local level, this also supports the need for more research to identify the range of impacts, as discussed in Chapter 6.

Evaluating the impact of advocacy

In addressing the challenges above, there are some important considerations. Focusing on what matters to advocacy partners is clearly important and, therefore, requires involving people with experience of compulsion and advocates in defining outcomes and criteria for assessing IMHA services. Being clear about the purpose of evaluating outcomes is critical and, as noted from the earlier discussion, different stakeholders and their organisations will have different motivations for wanting to understand the impact of IMHA services. Service users might frame the purpose of understanding impact in terms of reducing the number of people detained; IMHA services might frame it in terms of understanding whether there is a relationship between impact and the length of time spent with an individual partner, and commissioners in terms of service quality or cost effectiveness. These agendas are not mutually exclusive but, not least because of limited human and financial resources, it is important to develop a shared view of the purpose of evaluating impact. This will also shape the kind of information that will be sought.

The earlier discussion has also highlighted the importance of understanding whether and how IMHA has an impact on staff behaviour and ward culture. This could include service user assessments of staff attitudes and the extent to which they feel that their care and treatment is person centred, as well as initiatives to assess ward culture in terms of the understanding and support for advocacy. Finally, consideration should be given to evaluating short-term and long-term outcomes, and Table 8.2 illustrates this in terms of process outcomes and change outcomes, both of which contribute to quality of life outcomes.

TABLE 8.2 SHORT-TERM AND LONG-TERM IMPACTS OF INDEPENDENT MENTAL HEALTH ADVOCACY		
Outcomes	Short term	Long term
Process	Improved awareness of rights and understanding of the mental health system. Exercising rights and having a say in decision making. Service users are able to direct their own care meetings.	Ability to plan for self and keep well and live independently. Change in ward culture, enabling person-centred approaches and improvements in how service users are treated by mental health professionals. Increased accountability of mental health professionals.
Change	Increased self-confidence and self-esteem. Better able to self-advocate and negotiate care and treatment. Addressing issues affecting mental health.	Being able to sort out or access support to help with any issues that could affect independent living or mental health. Avoidance of compulsory admission or rehospitalisation.

Theory-driven approaches and logic modelling

Theory-driven approaches offer a way of linking the process and change outcomes, moving beyond narrow approaches to input–output evaluation (Miller 2011) to understand how a particular intervention or programme works. This starts with exploring the underlying assumptions about how an intervention (in this case advocacy) is meant to work (Anderson 2005). The evaluation focus then becomes an examination of the extent to which desired outcomes have been achieved with the inputs and outputs or activities of a project or service.

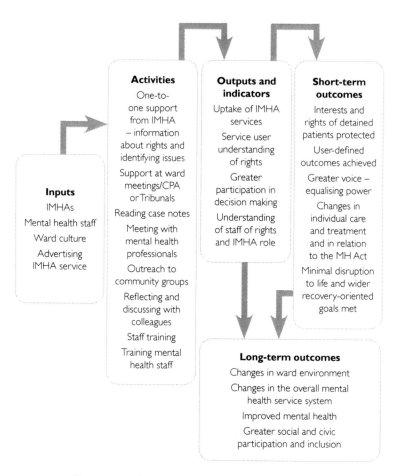

*Figure 8.2 A logic model for evaluating the impact
of independent mental health advocacy*

Adopting this approach brings different stakeholders (service users, carers, advocates, mental health staff, commissioners and others) together to define the endpoints that they want to reach and to explore the activities and processes required to achieve it. They can include defining soft outcomes, outcomes that arise on the way, and longer-term outcomes. Logic modelling is an example of a theory-driven approach and can help organisations develop greater clarity about what they are working to achieve (Miller 2011). Logic models can be constructed in a variety of ways, and Figure 8.2 provides a simple example for IMHA using the data collected during our study: logic models may be more detailed but in any event they reduce the complexity providing a heuristic to guide evaluation.

Eliciting and recording process and change outcomes

The previous section describes an overall approach within which different types of information can be collected. Here, we consider the different types of information and approaches, encompassing the different levels outlined in Figure 8.1 – individual, family and social, service and civic. In our study, we found a degree of consensus that the most appropriate measures should be based on measuring both process and change outcomes associated with the key role and purpose of IMHA – for example, qualifying patients' increased knowledge and understanding of their rights, a decrease in the number of unlawful detentions and an increase in the quality of appeals. Box 8.2 provides an example of the measures adopted by one advocacy service, following a telephone survey of former advocacy partners.

BOX 8.2 SIX PERSONAL OUTCOMES OF INSTRUCTED MENTAL HEALTH ADVOCACY INCLUDING IMHA

- The person using advocacy will feel they are making progress with the issue(s) they bring to advocacy.

- The person using advocacy will feel they are being heard/listened to more.

- The person using advocacy will feel they know more about their rights and options.

- The person using advocacy will feel they have more influence over decisions.

- The person using advocacy will feel better supported/ less distressed in relation to the issue(s) they brought to advocacy.

- The person using advocacy will feel more confident about dealing with the issue(s) they bring to advocacy.

(Source: Newbigging et al. 2012a, p.198)

This demonstrates an emphasis on process outcomes, although it would be possible to develop it further so that there was a stronger focus on the advocacy partner's satisfaction with achieving outcomes as they define them.

On the face of it, it appears relatively easy for advocacy services to evaluate whether advocacy partners' requests or aspirations have been fulfilled by matching what happened (actual outcome) with the initial request(s) (desired outcome). This approach is commonly used and is compatible with the person-centred principles of advocacy. For this to be useful, the information needs to be aggregated to build a comprehensive picture of the impact of IMHA services. There may, however, be initial difficulties in establishing what qualifying patients want because the context of compulsion may effectively 'silence' some people or lower their aspirations. Frameworks that provide a guide can be useful and also enable advocacy services to compare outcomes across different service users. An example of this approach is the 'I' statements developed by Think Local Act Personal (TLAP) in relation to service user-defined outcomes for adult social care, and more recently for mental health services (National Voices and TLAP NSUN 2014). Building on this, Table 8.3 provides a series of 'I' statements developed through the implementation project for IMHA services. This framework of 'I' statements provides a starting point for assessing the outcomes of IMHA against service user-defined goals, which broadly reflect the issues of autonomy, participation, care and recovery as identified in Chapter 5. Writing outcomes as 'I' statements is powerful because it is focused on the individuals using the services and reflects person-centred working, supporting the move to more personalised services in general.

TABLE 8.3 EXAMPLES OF 'I' STATEMENTS FOR EVALUATING IMHA SERVICES	
Outcome type	**Proposed outcome written as an 'I' statement**
Process	I know what my rights under the MH Act are and feel able to exercise them. I have a say in how decisions are made about my care, treatment and leave. I am treated with respect and dignity and my heritage and culture is understood and recognised as part of my recovery. I feel I have more control over my care and treatment. I understand how the mental health system works and how it affects me personally. If I raise complaints or concerns about a service these are taken seriously and acted upon, and I am told what has happened in response.
Change	I have moved to the least restrictive care in the earliest possible time for me, e.g. being discharged from a section. I feel my self-confidence and self-esteem has increased as a result of being able to voice my views. I feel I have greater control over managing my mental health, including in a crisis. I am able to get on with my life and be involved with people and activities that matter to me.

Methods for capturing this type of information could include questionnaires, interviews, online surveys and adopting specific question formats. Using Likert scales, which involve asking participants to circle or tick a value listed on a sliding scale (numbers, words or emoticons can be used), against statements like those in Table 8.3, can help increase accessibility of such methods. *Lost in Translation*, published by Action for Advocacy (2009), suggests a range of formats for presenting outcome statements and methods for rating.[1] Distance-travelled measurements or longitudinal

---

1   Available at: www.aqvx59.dsl.pipex.com/Lost_in_translation.pdf (accessed on 17 January 2015).

measures used at different time points are helpful in identifying any changes in an individual's situation that has occurred between initial access to an IMHA service and the last encounter (Action for Advocacy 2009). A baseline measurement is required and repeated at termination of the IMHA involvement and/or on being discharged from hospital – the comparison between the two enabling any impact to be identified. An example of this type of measure is the advocacy outcomes radar tool developed by the Gateshead Advocacy Information Network (GAIN), illustrated in Figure 8.3. GAIN worked with seven local advocacy projects and advocacy service users to develop a monitoring and evaluation framework in relation to advocacy outcomes relating to Putting People First (Department of Health 2007). Advocates found that introducing the outcome radar sparked useful conversations about the service users' wider life, their independence, sense of choice, etc. and supported advocates to reflect on their own practice too (Broadbridge 2014).

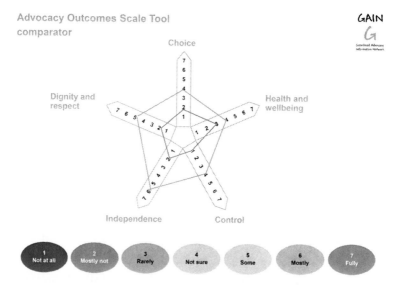

Figure 8.3 Gateshead Advocacy Information Network advocacy outcomes radar tool (Source: Gateshead Advocacy Information Network – Broadbridge 2012)

Collecting qualitative information through interviews, focus groups or advocacy partners keeping diaries, creative writing or through visual material such as photo diaries and drawings will enable more detailed and nuanced evaluation of the impact of IMHA services (SCIE/UCLan 2015). Individual-level information will need collating and analysing to identify common themes and important differences in experiences of partners from different backgrounds, in different circumstances.

Not all advocacy partners may be willing to participate in providing feedback and, therefore, consideration needs to be given to making this as accessible and attractive as possible, for example by linking to existing group or community activities. Over-reliance on written formats may mean that people who are less literate will not complete them without support. The question of who undertakes the evaluation, whether this is routinely done in-house through the IMHA service or commissioned from an independent body, for example a service user organisation, is also an important consideration, with the latter likely to be preferred. In our implementation project, service users promoted the use of online methods (e.g. Survey Monkey surveys) which could be completed anonymously and at the service user's own pace. This would require access to computers on wards, as well as in hospital café facilities, and support from peers or volunteers if people lack computer literacy skills or confidence. The extent to which quantitative data is considered – for example, in relation to demographic characteristics, detention rates and numbers of appeals – is also worth considering, although the absence of qualitative data, for example on the quality of appeals, may render this difficult to interpret. The resolution of these issues will be determined by clarity about the objectives of the evaluation, as well as practical support to implement the desired approach.

Evaluating changes in professional behaviour and organisational culture will prove more challenging, although they provide an interesting focus for research. In our study, several service users and some mental health staff identified how the presence of IMHAs on the ward and in various meetings acted as an important safeguard against poor practice and as such was potentially a force for changing practice by opening up staff attitudes and behaviour and the ward culture to external scrutiny. Such outcomes will be reflected in service user evaluations of the extent to which they have been listened to, participated in decision making, or treated with care and compassion. An audit of case notes and CPA plans could also reveal the extent to which the IMHA leads to changes in specific treatment and support or overall approach, although in our study IMHA involvement appeared to be rarely recorded. Positive changes in staff behaviour and ward culture may be the result of other initiatives, for example introducing recovery-oriented practice or peer support. This reinforces the need for service users', as well as staff and carers', reflections on the ward culture and their assessment of the contribution of IMHA services. Overall, the impact of advocacy at this level is going to be more difficult to capture within routine monitoring and evaluation of services, and is likely a more long-term impact, but should form the basis for future research using observational methods.

Finally, the extent to which service users are achieving wider recovery goals should be a focus for ongoing evaluation, both at an individual and service level. IMHAs are one element of enabling service users to improve their overall situation, and arguably dependent on the service ethos for achieving this. Different methods are used for this purpose, and the recovery star is commonly used.[2]

Cost effectiveness

If one of the outcomes from IMHA provision is that people receive a more appropriate service, informed by what they want and consistent with their personal goals, then it seems likely that IMHA provision will both be cost effective and provide a social return on the investment (SROI). SROI is being used by advocacy projects to demonstrate the benefits of advocacy, typically on an individual basis, which commissioners can find helpful

---

2   Available at www.outcomesstar.org.uk/mental-health (accessed on 26 January 2015).

in understanding the nature and benefits of IMHA services (Newbigging *et al.* 2012a). Macadam *et al.* (2013) identified that few studies had considered cost effectiveness and, in part, this reflects difficulties in identifying outcomes and costs (Bauer *et al.* 2013). In our study, we found that routine monitoring of activity and uptake of IMHA services was being undertaken, but the lack of aggregated data on outcomes and costs made it difficult to establish cost effectiveness. Nevertheless, this was highlighted as important to understand and likely to be a future direction for research and local evaluation of services. An example of how this might be approached is provided by an evaluation of the cost effectiveness of advocacy for parents with learning disabilities (Bauer *et al.* 2013). The research team used a questionnaire to capture data on:

- inputs – number of staff employed, salary ranges, extent of training and supervision, average travelling time, size of caseloads, number and mean duration of meetings, mean duration of time spent on preparation and the number and type of referrals or signposting to other interventions

- outputs and outcomes – reasons for the referral, point at which advocates became involved, outcomes achieved through the advocacy intervention and activities that the advocacy projects believed were linked to advocacy and activities or procedures that the projects believed had been prevented as a result of advocacy interventions. (p.6)

From this, costs per hour and case were calculated and the main net benefit across cases, cost savings of advocacy, main net benefit of advocacy, the economic value of reduced quality of life impairments and productivity gains of parents were estimated. The results showed that costs and benefits varied greatly from case to case, and the research team concluded that it was difficult to draw generalisable conclusions based on a small number of cases. However, their tentative findings did indicate that investment in advocacy for this particular group could reduce costs in the short term and bring benefits in terms of savings from a wider public sector perspective and quality of life improvements.

The cost effectiveness of IMHA has yet to be demonstrated, but a promising line of inquiry would be to consider its impact on expenditure on in-patient care (i.e. reducing length of stays, preventing readmission) and personal outcomes in terms of quality of life (i.e. improved confidence, health and well-being).

Conclusions

The importance of demonstrating that IMHA, indeed any advocacy, is making a difference to individuals and communities is undisputed. The increasing emphasis on outcomes-focused commissioning has added impetus to the need to address the challenges of evaluating the effectiveness, as well as the quality, of advocacy services, with the self-evident worth of advocacy no longer being sufficient to guarantee its continued survival (Action for Advocacy 2009). The impact and outcomes of advocacy are inherently difficult to measure, and this is reflected in the lack of evidence highlighted by our research review in Chapter 6. In relation to IMHA, a key benefit experienced by service users, and acknowledged by others, is an increase in their understanding of rights under the legislation and, from the service users' perspective, greater understanding of their situation. Bound up with an important commitment towards service user empowerment, IMHAs ensure that the service user's voice does not go unheard.

There is, however, a concern that IMHA services can serve to bolster the status quo through placating people subject to compulsion whilst not achieving a tangible change in their situation (McKeown et al. 2013). On the other hand, reports of minimal or no impact may reflect a lack of appreciation or lack of knowledge about what constitutes a recognisable outcome of advocacy. Furthermore, service users may not necessarily always credit advocacy with the outcome, believing they would have achieved the change without the advocate's involvement. The issue the service user wanted help with was perhaps something the IMHA could not support them to achieve immediately, e.g. getting out of hospital, or the service user is aware that they could benefit from some support (e.g. in a ward round or Tribunal) and that an advocate could possibly help, but has not asked for that kind of help from the advocate. There are various circumstances where the IMHA service alone might have little impact in terms of what the individual wants or on the social circumstances of a person's life. Theory of change models can help disentangle some of these issues and provide a framework for understanding the relationship between the process of advocacy and outcomes achieved.

Agreed outcome statements developed by a range of stakeholders, importantly inclusive of service users, is crucial for monitoring and evaluation. Utilising an 'I' statement format can be very powerful and convey the important impacts from a service user perspective. Different stakeholders may have different outcome needs, but unless service users are involved in the development of agreed outcomes and measurement tools, any impact due to IMHA intervention is likely to be lessened or reduced to a tick box exercise. On paper, a service may appear to offer high-quality provision, but if it doesn't make a positive difference to the experiences and eventual recovery of the individual concerned then it becomes meaningless (Stewart and MacIntyre 2013), and fails the original aspirations of the MH Act 2007. The challenge of evaluating the impact of advocacy is, therefore, an important one in which service users, advocacy services, commissioners and researchers need to engage.

REFLECTIVE EXERCISES

1. Make a list of the key challenges advocacy services face in measuring the difference IMHA services make in the lives of advocacy partners, and how you think these could be overcome.

2. What impacts do you think IMHA services can achieve for people using them?

3. Put yourself in the shoes of a service user, a carer, a staff member (e.g. mental health nurse or AMHP and a commissioner – what advocacy outcomes might each of these be interested in? Make four columns and list the likely outcomes of IMHA services that might be sought by each group.

4. How would you go about evaluating the process and change outcomes of advocacy?

Chapter 9

DOING INDEPENDENT MENTAL HEALTH ADVOCACY WELL

Values, Knowledge and Skills

Introduction

In this chapter we turn our attention to highlighting the values, knowledge base and skills required to ensure effective IMHA practice. We have written this chapter primarily from a service user perspective, drawing on our first-hand experience alongside data from interviews with 90 qualifying patients who participated in our research. We also refer to the general literature on independent advocacy, in particular the knowledge and skills outlined in the national Certificate in Independent Advocacy, the need for which was signalled by the development of statutory forms of advocacy. If advocates are to genuinely work in partnership with service users, the skill set needed includes good skills in relationship building, communication and listening, and they need to operate from a strong values base that emphasises user-focused practice and a social justice approach. Figure 9.1 summarises these tripartite elements.

Before looking at each of these in turn, we assert our view that true 'professionalism' in advocacy means integrating appropriate values, knowledge and skills, with relationship building a key element. In developing an advocacy partnership, building a good relationship should be regarded as central, and the fact that this is essentially a partisan relationship, unambiguously on the side of the advocacy partner, is not antithetical to professionalism. When writing about doing advocacy well we also take into consideration that IMHAs have to operate within a complex multi-disciplinary system, and this has a bearing upon the knowledge and skills required of them to advocate effectively for service users.

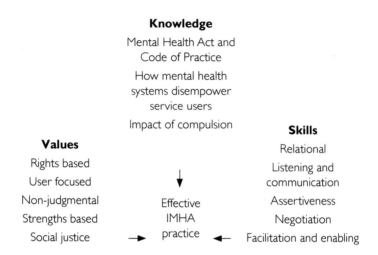

Figure 9.1 Elements of effective IMHA practice

Values and principles for effective practice

At the time of detention the world of the service user feels a very unsafe place, both the world left outside and the world of the hospital ward. IMHAs need to allow themselves to 'live' these emotions with the service user in a managed way, maintaining safety: both their own and that of the service user. It is only through genuine empathy and rapport that the advocate can enable partners to develop self-esteem and confidence to move from that lonely place they can be locked into, often literally. There are established common values or ethical codes underlying best practice in the 'helping professions' such as social work and nursing that are readily transposed into consideration of core values for IMHA practice. Specifically, these include treating people with respect and promoting their dignity, upholding their rights, being non-judgmental person focused, and adopting a social justice approach.

Rights-focused approach

Belief in the inherent worth and respect for the dignity of all human beings is a fundamental principle sustaining advocacy practice. This is supported by legislation in accordance with universal rights charters, for example the United Nations Declaration of Human Rights (1948). Adopting such rights-based practice goes some way to addressing the obvious power imbalances between mental health professionals and service users. Advocates need to be aware that they too will have an impact on the power dynamics, for better or worse. Similarly, health and social work professionals need to be aware of the limitations of their claims to an advocacy role and acting in people's 'best interests' (Bateman 2000; Brandon and Brandon 2000): see Chapter 11.

Maintaining respect for the dignity of service users also engenders a strengths-based perspective to advocacy practice, which ultimately will develop the resilience, confidence and capability of service users. In the crisis of compulsory admission, service users receive negative messages about themselves that have the potential to reinforce stereotyping and stigmatising identities, and can result in people feeling worthless or that their viewpoint is invalid. It is imperative, therefore, that IMHAs support partners to regain a sense of self-worth in as short a time as possible. While it may seem that this is outside the advocate's remit, without supporting partners' self-esteem, little positive movement can be made in the advocacy partnership, or indeed in service users' lives. Indeed, such efforts go to the heart of aspirations to support people to be able to speak for themselves.

IMHAs need to respect the rights of individuals to self-determination and participation in decision making. These factors are critical to IMHA as distinct from advocacy in the 'best interests' of the person, where a professional such as a nurse or social worker acts on someone's behalf, bringing to bear their professional knowledge and understanding of the situation (Bateman 2000; Dalrymple and Boylan 2013; Jugessur and Iles 2009). Independent advocacy should also be distinguished from advice giving, though the government's recent post-legislative scrutiny of the MH Act 2007 (House of Commons 2013) muddies the waters somewhat in recommending extending the IMHA role to include advice giving. Legal representation will differ from the IMHA service in this respect, engaging as it does with giving legal advice and/or representing the best interests of the service user.

User-focused/person-centred approach

The importance of adopting a user-focused or person-centred approach cannot be overstated. It is critical that the IMHA is able to relate to a person's unique reality and perceptions. This may necessitate suspending disbelief and including previously unshared perceptions of reality and cognitive viewpoints. So many times mental health service users are dismissed as fantasists who are delusional or 'lacking insight'. It is vital for the IMHA to recognise that the service user's story may include near and distant experiences which have meaning for them but which may be out of context and framed in an unusual way. One service user sums up this ability as an IMHA being able to:

> speak lucidly and with empathy [and] not just sympathetic but to put yourself in the, not the mind because we're supposed to be so ill, but to put yourself in the feelings of the patient and speak accordingly for the patient. (Service user quoted in Newbigging *et al.* 2012a, p.124)

Not judging is a fundamental requirement for effective advocacy. However, subjectivity inevitably informs judgments and it is important that the IMHA always acknowledges their personal prejudices and reflects on them to minimise any effect on practice. An ability to work in a non-judgmental and user-focused way therefore behoves advocates to start from where the service user is currently (Lawton 2006). When the IMHA suspends disbelief, they will be able to hear the hidden and deeper meaning in the service user's account, which can play such an important part in the planning and making of an effective advocacy case, as the following advocate observes:

> He told me he had no red blood cells. This was obviously impossible. He would be dead and not standing in front

of me. However, this was what he was experiencing. He felt very tired, as if his red blood cells had all been killed off. He was very distressed. He had informed medical staff and they had told him not to be silly, it was just part of his mental illness and the tablets would help him. After some discussion I realised he was referring to the side effects of his medication. We spoke with his doctor who reduced his dosage and his experience went away. (Unpublished work by Kaaren Cruse)

An ethical dilemma often exists for the IMHA working betwixt the competing agendas of professionals and service users. Put another way, how does the IMHA manage the process so that they remain focused on the needs and wants of the advocacy partner which may conflict with professionals' best interests concerns? The skills identified later in this chapter should help IMHAs to navigate such challenges, staying with the service user's agenda while avoiding privileging the 'best interests' preference of the professional agenda. As a result, advocates can sometimes be viewed by professionals as naïve and as lacking in understanding of the service user's condition. Essentially, though, as one advocate comments, the IMHA role is about ensuring the service user's voice is heard, and should always be the primary focus of their work:

> The staff think I don't understand mental illness because I work with someone who hears voices. He believes they are helping him as they say kind things and he thinks they are his spirit guides. I just accept his voices and talk to him about options. I have to be very calm, and work hard to enable staff to listen to his views. (Unpublished work by Kaaren Cruse)

Social justice approach

Advocacy practice that is empowering means not only working at the level of the individual, but also involves operating within a complex mental health system, challenging anti-oppressive practice and ensuring the collective as well as individual voice of service users is heard. IMHAs need to exercise their duty and authority, individually and collectively, to challenge conditions that contribute to social exclusion, stigmatisation, stereotyping and the discrimination and oppression of people with mental health problems – thus ultimately promoting a more inclusive attitude in society. The IMHA role is pivotal to enhancing quality of life for mental health service users when they are faced with deprivation of their liberty or enforced treatments.

It may be that scarce resources limit the capacity of mental health services to deliver good-quality care and positive outcomes for service users, potentially infringing rights, as discussed in Chapter 4. IMHAs need to disentangle whether decisions promote the well-being of service users, or if they actually reflect resource shortfalls. Proper attention to diverse needs and social justice aspirations can be severely impeded when faced with financial constraints. IMHAs need to support service users to challenge decisions resulting in inadequate service provision that is unfairly biased by resource shortfalls.

Knowledge base

There are differing viewpoints about the knowledge of mental health required of IMHAs. We argue that, essentially, IMHAs need to have a sound knowledge of the Mental Health Act and of service users' rights under this law, and they need to understand what the experience of compulsion is like and the profound impact this can have on a person's life (see Chapter 5 and also Berg-Cross *et al.* 2011).

Mental health law

As detailed in Chapter 4, the Code of Practice and supporting guidance outlines the IMHA role in supporting qualifying patients to articulate their views, to access information and to participate as fully as possible in discussions and decision making relevant to them. In order to fulfil this role, IMHAs therefore need to be knowledgeable and up to date about mental health law as it relates to qualifying patients. They need to understand people's rights and entitlements under this law including their rights to appeal, to complain, to access information, to change their medication and to apply for leave and discharge. IMHAs need to be able to apply and communicate this information in accessible ways to a diverse range of qualifying patients, taking account of different communication capabilities or needs.

The knowledge required of an IMHA is to a large extent defined by the way the role is legislated for in the MH Act 2007 and detailed in the Code of Practice (Department of Health 2015), and this is reflected in the learning objectives of the national IMHA course (see Box 9.1). During introduction of the IMHA role, a framework for training and standards was developed, and an accredited City and Guilds Certificate is now delivered in five modules, comprising a specialist unit (306) in IMHA. Initially, preparation for the IMHA role was delivered by the Department of Health training team and consisted of four days, which could then be topped up with the City and Guilds modules, thus amounting to the full Certificate in Independent Advocacy. This training is now delivered by a number of organisations across England.

BOX 9.1 OUTLINE OF THE CITY AND GUILDS CERTIFICATE IN INDEPENDENT ADVOCACY

The Level 3 Certificate in Independent Advocacy is a Qualification Credit Framework (QCF) competency-based qualification. This means that those registering for it must demonstrate their skills and knowledge in undertaking a range of advocacy-specific activities in their workplace. The qualification is made up of four core units which are assessed at Level 3 and focus on the core requirements for advocacy:

- Unit 301: Purpose and principles of independent advocacy.

- Unit 302: Providing independent advocacy support.

- Unit 303: Maintaining the independent advocacy relationship.

- Unit 304: Understanding the social context of independent advocacy.

Candidates must also complete their chosen option from a range of pathway units, including Unit 306 for IMHA, which are assessed at Level 4.

The Level 4 qualification covers the basic principles and purpose of independent advocacy, how to effectively respond to the advocacy needs of different groups of people and, with the Diploma, how to make decisions on behalf of individuals subject to Deprivation of Liberty Safeguards.

Completion can take six months to one year full time or one to two years part time and includes the following areas of assessment: direct observation of work-based activity, expert witness, work products, professional discussion, reflective accounts and questions by the assessor.

Modules covered are the introduction to the IMHA role, the framework of legislation for IMHAs, the qualifying patient and the mental health system, effective IMHA practice and principles, and skills for effective IMHA practice.

Other specialist modules can also be added to Level 4, including providing IMCA, providing Deprivation of Liberty Safeguards and mental capacity legislation for the independent advocacy role.

(Sources: National Mental Health Development Unit 2009b; Welsh Government, City and Guilds London Institute and Advocacy Training, Consultation and Supervision 2008.)[1]

As our study found, understanding rights and having access to information about these is empowering in itself, especially if you have been sectioned for the first time and are feeling vulnerable, isolated and lost. In addition, IMHAs clearly need to understand

---

1   Specifically relevant to the Welsh context.

the mechanisms for appeal under the law, for example the right to a Tribunal or a Manager's Hearing, and other rights, if they are to effectively support service users to access them. The needs of individual service users requesting IMHA support will determine what is required in any particular situation, so that the advocate always remains true to respecting and working to the wishes of the service user, holding the ultimate goal of self-advocacy in mind.

Experiences of compulsion and mental health services

We argued in Part 1 that it is vital that IMHAs have some understanding of the different discourses around mental health and distress, and we further contend that it is important they are familiar with the literature around direct experiences of compulsion (see Chapter 5). In other words, they need to understand how the physical environment of a locked ward can impact on an individual, or what it feels like to have your freedom curtailed in the environment of your home. Damage to identity can be an aspect of the causation, experience and continuation of mental health problems. Of equal or even greater significance is the loss of identity on finding yourself in the psychiatric system, particularly when you are an in-patient. Personal identifiers such as those denoting family or job role and associated social status can be submerged by the all-consuming identity of the 'psychiatric patient' or, worse still, under the label of a diagnosed disorder. Thus, mental health service users' experiences become pathologised and dehumanised. Having some understanding of how it feels to be detained, therefore, is a critical part of the knowledge base IMHAs need in order to practise effectively (Ridley and Hunter 2013; Russo and Wallcraft 2011). There is also a case – founded similarly on the belief that possessing knowledge offsets feelings of powerlessness and empowers service users – that IMHAs should possess some working knowledge of medical understandings and terminology relating to diagnoses in order to increase their effectiveness. In our study, some service users, along with some mental health staff, considered this important, as one service user explains:

> I am continuously dealing with doctors and I talk at their
> level and I have that understanding and therefore I remain at
> that level and to actually engage with somebody who is not
> understanding that, it is difficult for me. Especially when I'm
> unwell…it took a lot of effort for me to, to put it into crystal
> clear… I have to do all the explanation…and the explanation
> wore me out. (Service user quoted in Newbigging *et al.* 2012a,
> p.187)

The value of having some understanding of medical terminology
is not the same as accepting its legitimacy, however. Many service
users find mental health staff's use of jargon to be off-putting and
mystifying, and that it reinforces prevailing power imbalances
between professionals and service users. As a result, they point
to the importance of the IMHA role in helping to dismantle and
challenge the status quo:

> [IMHAs are] very down to earth and they don't come out
> with all the mumbo jumbo speak, you know they talk in plain
> English… I think they're quite friendly, open and friendly.
> It didn't appear officious because you can be put off people
> who talk with all this new jargon and yeah, and people don't
> understand it. (Service user quoted in Newbigging *et al.*
> 2012a, p.131)

IMHAs need to have some understanding of, and/or be able to
research, the terms and jargon used by mental health staff when
service users find these difficult to understand and staff do not
explain them clearly. They need to know how to help service users
look for information they want, for instance about mental health
diagnoses, the impact of treatments or particular drugs on the
individual and so on, but they also need to know that their role
is to facilitate communication between service users and mental
health staff who themselves have a duty to inform about care
and treatment and to involve service users in decisions. IMHAs'
strategy therefore should be to challenge mental health service
staff to make the language they use in diagnosing mental health
problems and treatment decisions crystal clear. Only in this way

will the power and control in these situations come anywhere near to being more democratic.

Skill set needed by IMHAs

For IMHAs to practise effectively they need to use a range of skills. These are often identified as core skills in communication and listening, assertiveness and negotiation (Action for Advocacy 2012; Bateman 2000; Townsley *et al.* 2009). In addition, relationship building is paramount, alongside the ability to act independently (Brooke 2002; Palmer *et al.* 2012). Being 'diplomatic' with staff – that is, being assertive enough to understand different perspectives whilst remaining person centred – is felt by advocates to lead to better outcomes for service users (Palmer *et al.* 2012, p.77). Our work suggests that in order to operate in complex environments, and keep service users' needs to the forefront, IMHAs need to develop strong relationship-building skills, as well as skills in communication and listening, and other interpersonal skills, particularly assertiveness, facilitation and negotiation.

Relationship-building skills

Skills in building relationships with qualifying patients, and also with a range of mental health service staff and others, lie at the heart of the IMHA role. Effective IMHA services act to support and enable service users to be involved in decision making and ensure that the service user voice is heard. Developing meaningful and trusting relationships with service users is therefore critical. The relationship aspect is often cited as pivotal to effective advocacy intervention. As we discuss in the previous chapter, even when desired outcomes or aspirations are not met through the advocacy partnership, service users will highlight positive impacts arising from the relationship with an advocate, both in terms of having someone who is on their side who listens to their views, and how this affects interactions with professionals (as discussed in Chapter 8; see also Townsley *et al.* 2009).

The skill of relationship building is based on a number of qualities and attributes that have been highlighted over the years in humanistic psychology, as discussed in Chapter 2. It almost goes without saying that the ability to develop trust is essential (Palmer *et al.* 2012), and can depend on the ability of advocates to successfully utilise a range of interpersonal skills. This can be especially significant for someone who is detained, particularly if for the first time, and they don't know what to expect or who to trust:

> I was given the number of the IMHA but didn't like to call. Everyone could hear my call including the nurses. I didn't know who I was talking to, they could be anyone, they could be agents for staff. I was struggling with paranoia and couldn't trust no-one, I felt very alone and frightened. I watched the IMHA lady come on to the ward, listened to what others said about her. After several weeks I talked with her, a few days after I told her about what was happening to me. She listened, I felt I didn't have to be alone, she would help me. She liked me... She said she could help, she didn't say that was the illness talking. (Service user quoted in Newbigging *et al.* 2012a p.124)

Relationships grounded in trust also need an environment of genuineness, warmth, acceptance and empathy (Rogers 1967). Having a shared identity as a service user or a member of a similar BAME community can facilitate this, as we explore in Chapter 10. Adopting a person-focused and non-judgmental approach, the IMHA also needs to develop skills in tackling barriers to relationships in complex situations (Ruch, Turney and Ward 2010). Building relationships that are beneficial for service users also means being heard by mental health professionals involved in care and treatment (Featherstone and Fraser 2012; Lawton 2006). IMHAs therefore need to use different strategies to engage with mental health service staff in a range of settings, and to be as skilled in building these relationships as they are in relating to different service users.

Communication and listening skills

Effective relationships with qualifying patients and professionals at all levels require that IMHAs have good communication and listening skills (Bateman 2000). They need to use appropriate communication methods to meet the needs of individuals, for example those with hearing impairments, those whose first language is not English or those with learning disabilities. It is also important that they communicate their role clearly to professionals. As in our study, service users commonly cite the key importance of listening skills when asked what makes a good IMHA:

> A good listener, that's all you really need. Half the time all you need is someone to listen to you, you know and not going yeah, yeah, yeah no bother, you know, all you need is someone that is going to listen to you. (Service user quoted in Newbigging et al. 2012a, p.124)

Good communication skills therefore will include active listening skills and effective adaptation of communication styles to suit the audience (including employing user-friendly language), and the ability to suspend disbelief and attune to and support the service user's articulation of their experiences or accurately represent their views if requested to do so. Good listening skills ensure that advocates communicate effectively, do not impose their interpretation of events (Bateman 2000) and that the voice of the user is heard. IMHAs will need to be able to adapt and articulate information and key messages in ways that can be assimilated and understood by the diverse range of qualifying patients eligible for IMHA (Lawton 2006), and work in culturally sensitive ways (Fazil et al. 2004; Newbigging and McKeown 2007; Newbigging et al. 2013). Additionally, advocates will need to communicate service users' viewpoints to mental health service staff in ways that they can understand while remaining faithful to what the service user wants.

Facilitation and enabling skills

As compulsory detention is a time of great uncertainty for service users whose world has often been turned upside down, and as they try to make sense of what seems completely meaningless, IMHAs need to work alongside and support them to articulate their views and to be involved in decision making. It will be important, therefore, that IMHAs are skilled facilitators and enablers, able to support service users through the complexities of process, situation and feelings, and above all the loss of liberty and control over their lives, on a journey to self-advocacy and recovery.

Assertiveness skills

To act in a person-focused way, supporting the service user's priorities, IMHAs will need to have good assertiveness skills. In the mental health context, this means standing up for service users' rights, expressing their views and feelings in direct, honest and appropriate ways. This also involves respecting the thoughts, feelings and beliefs of others involved in the process so that views are conveyed in a way that does not compromise the validity of the service user's perspective, nor impact negatively on their treatment.

Negotiation skills

To have good negotiation skills is an important part of the skill set required of IMHAs, as these are needed in working with and supporting service users to understand and exercise their right to be involved and heard in decision-making forums such as Tribunals, Manager's Hearings, CPA meetings and so on. Underpinning negotiation skills are a range of other skills such as critical analytical skills, which will enable IMHAs to support service users to consider all options in decision making, respecting that ultimately it will be up to the service user what they want to do. IMHAs sometimes need to signpost qualifying patients to people and other services or work in partnership with community organisations that have a developed understanding of the relevant social and cultural contexts of a person's life.

Conclusions

In this chapter we have argued that effective IMHA practice and the delivery of quality IMHA services depend critically upon IMHAs acting from the right value base, having knowledge and understanding, and applying this through a range of practice skills. In particular, we have stressed the importance of advocacy practice based on sound user-led values and principles. That is, practice that is rights based, person focused and in pursuit of social justice goals. Such values are the foundation and should be the drivers of good practice. As well as being knowledgeable about the legislation and how it relates to qualifying patients, IMHAs should have some knowledge of what service users say about the experience of being detained under a section, and of the ways that the mental health system disempowers service users. The complex skill set required includes relationship building and interpersonal skills so that IMHAs communicate effectively with the diverse range of qualifying patients, as well as effectively representing their wishes in negotiation with mental health service staff and in a range of settings such as Tribunals and CPA meetings.

The need for training and supervision to skill up advocates for effective interventions is cited in the majority of research carried out on advocacy practice. In addition it is included in the government's post-legislative scrutiny of the Mental Health Act 2007 (House of Commons 2013). This training should involve the use of person-focused approaches, as well as the inclusion of service users' expertise. People with mental health problems are not a homogeneous group. IMHAs therefore need the knowledge and skills to be able to respond to diverse cultural, communication and other needs. As people with mental health problems are more likely to experience barriers to accessing information and support (Butters, Webster and Hill 2010), it is vital that they are involved in developing training programmes to enable the delivery of effective IMHA interventions. Finally, to ensure that knowledge and skills developed through training are used, and further development needs identified, regular supervision is essential.

REFLECTIVE EXERCISES

What follows is a powerful statement from one service user's perspective about what they would like from an IMHA. Read the statement and then consider the questions below, relating to it and the issues of the chapter:

What I would want from an IMHA – A service user's perspective

I would be in need of support for advocating against legal processes around compulsory detention and imposed coercive treatments. Therefore it would be essential for the IMHA to have a working knowledge of the MH Act. You may consider it would be in my interest if the IMHA knew about disorders, diagnoses and treatments, but it is my view that this knowledge is of little use, as in the particular situation of compulsory detention questioning of medical decisions isn't palatable to the medical professionals who hold the power and thus does not influence them to revise their opinions. The knowledge I would want the IMHA to have would give them particular expertise to challenge independently the professional power differential. I believe negotiating involving diagnosis, conditions and treatment further pathologises the individual and the conversation stays within the domain of the professional, increasing their power. Moreover, the IMHA could get too close to the

professional and further away from the service user.
Furthermore there is a danger that the IMHA could move
into the area of advice if medical professionalisation of
their role occurs. I firmly believe that advice giving should
not be part of the toolkit of the IMHA in the advocacy
relationship. If the wrong advice is given there could be
implications such as issues of liability. There is also the
danger that the IMHA could be disrespected by medical
professionals for having only a perfunctory knowledge of
medical matters.

---

1. Do you agree with the service user's assessment of what is needed to be an effective IMHA in this case?

2. Can you think of any situations where this approach wouldn't be as effective, and why?

3. List the practical implications of implementing an approach that emphasises the importance of values, knowledge and skills as discussed in the chapter, for example for the training and support of IMHAs.

4. Consider the ways in which IMHAs can work to promote self-advocacy. Can you identify any local examples of advocacy services working in this way?

Chapter 10

ONE SIZE FITS ALL?

Meeting Diverse Needs

Introduction

Social justice and equity are important considerations for the organisation and practice of appropriate advocacy services, just as they are for wider health and social care services. The terms inequality and inequity are often used interchangeably, as we do in this chapter. However, in general, inequality is used to refer to the condition of being unequal and commonly used in a UK context to capture a sense of disadvantage and unfairness.[1] Inequity is a more precise term and includes a judgment that this inequality is unfair and unjust and used to refer to differences in treatment of groups that are avoidable. Mental health services have a chequered history in their dealings with diversity issues, and in this chapter we explore this in relation to IMHA services and the extent to which its introduction has promoted equity.

We return to the theme of power and powerlessness that we discussed in Chapter 1 and expanded in subsequent chapters, and briefly explore how oppression and the exercise of power and control impact on people from diverse communities. This is well-documented in relation to the use of the MH Act for people from specific BAME backgrounds, notably people of African and African Caribbean heritage, who are more likely to be detained under the MH Act than those from White populations (CQC 2011). IMHA services can contribute to the process of resolving some of these problems but need to address equality and diversity issues in their own practice. This will include understanding the nature and impact of likely discrimination,

---

1   The term disparity is also used, particularly in a US context.

engaging with different conceptions of advocacy, exploring the implications for organisational design and delivery as well as the role of specialist advocates, and working in partnership with community organisations with specialist knowledge. Ultimately, what is provided will reflect the quality of commissioning and the decisions that are subsequently made about which organisations are best placed to deliver IMHA services, and we discuss the advantages and disadvantages of different arrangements.

Power and inequalities in mental health services

The term 'power' is often used somewhat loosely and we pause now to consider more nuanced theorising about the nature of power (Lukes 2005; first published 1974). Lukes (2005) distinguishes three dimensions or faces of power. The first 'involves a focus on behaviours in the making of decisions on issues over which there is an observable conflict of interests' (Lukes 2005, p.19). The framing of statutory advocacy as a mechanism for asserting the interests of service users, which can be in conflict with those of others, could be interpreted in this way.

Two- and three-dimensional power refers to more covert, possibly unconscious sources of power (Masterson and Owen 2006). A two-dimensional view of power considers the ways in which decisions are prevented from being taken as a result of an observable conflict of (subjective) interests (Lukes 2005). An example would be mental health professionals setting the agenda, and Masterson and Owen (2006) posit that the medical model applied to mental illness is an example of exercising this type of power. Other examples include excluding certain groups from research into mental health because of practical concerns about communication or capacity, or designing an advocacy service that responds to the needs of the majority and effectively ignores those of the minority.

A clear example of how limiting our analysis to a one- or two-dimensional view of power is insufficient can be seen in the experience of people from BAME communities in relation to the mental health system. Well documented elsewhere (see for example Fanon 1952, 2008; Fernando 2010; Keating 2007; Keating and Robertson 2004), the experience of the mental health system for people from BAME communities demonstrates the wider social inequities being played out through the mental health system.

People from African and Caribbean communities are more likely to be detained under the MH Act (CQC 2011), to be readmitted within a year (Priebe *et al.* 2009), to be placed in seclusion, to stay in hospital longer – and to have worse outcomes and negative experiences than people who form the majority community (Morgan 2012). Detained patients from BAME communities are also more likely to be subject to the overuse of medication and low use of psychological therapies (CQC 2011; NHS Information Centre 2011), compounding inequalities in outcomes and life chances.

A three-dimensional view of power goes further to suggest that social and/or institutional forces have a bearing on which issues are identified and, thus, legitimated (Lukes 2005). Kalathil and Faulkner (2015) thus argue that psychiatry and psychology have been complicit in the ways in which 'the pathologisation of the anger and disaffection among black communities, coupled with the racialised stereotype "big, black and dangerous", continue to colour psychiatric diagnosis in western societies with large populations of BAME communities' (p.23). From this perspective, power may be 'exercised by the manipulation of roles and identities so that certain groups may accept certain situations without conflict' (Masterson and Owens 2006, p.21), although there has been an extensive critique of mental health services and the treatment of BAME communities by BAME activists and communities.

From historical accounts we learn that social forces have played a key role in marginalising particular groups, and that the result is embedded in knowledge production[2] and rendered throughout institutional behaviours and norms. For people from BAME communities, the experience of the mental health system is associated with the legacy of slavery and colonialism, in which one race subjugated another.[3]

As Sadd (2014, p.50) observes:

> There are deep rooted similarities between colonialism and the psychiatric system. Both blighted my life for many years and would continue to do so if I had not become aware of the connections – the former caused it and the latter prolonged it. With and without physical slavery, races were made subjects of the ruling nations under the harsh experience of colonialism. This subjugation debilitated many peoples and nations historically, and continues to do so, through depriving them of their identity, which in turn impacts on their self-esteem and self-worth. People were at best infantilized or at worst demonized by the oppressors. Historically the psychiatric system has replicated the systems and structures of the colonial system, demonizing and infantilizing service users as it saw fit. Furthermore, despite attempts to liberalise the mental health system it is not hard to imagine why there is such distrust in it from BAME communities.

This critique represents a challenge to the current scaling up of mental health services based on approaches and models developed in high-income countries to low- and middle-income

---

2   A recent example is highlighted by Kalathil and Faulkner (2015) in their critique of a much lauded report produced by the British Psychological Society, arguing for multiple meanings of psychosis (Cooke 2014), but which ignored multiple viewpoints and scholarship relating to racialized experiencing and discrimination and psychiatry and psychology.

3   See, for example, Cartwright's (1851) *Diseases and Peculiarities of the Negro Race* for an insight into the historical context and the ways in which slavery was seen as benefiting the mental health of the enslaved and how medical conditions were fabricated to explain behaviour which was dysfunctional to the smooth efficiency of the plantations, for example behaviour such as running away.

services, placing alternative meanings, forms of support and the role of the local context, including knowledge and skills, in jeopardy (White and Sashidharan 2014).

Whilst we have focused on people from BAME communities, these forces are evident for other groups for whom discrimination and perpetuation of disadvantage through mental health services are a real risk, including people with sensory impairments, learning disabilities or other disabilities; older people or children and young people; women;[4] and lesbian, gay, bisexual and transgender people.[5] As we have argued, the epistemic injustices can be writ large for people from these groups. Empowerment thus takes on a particular complexion for marginalised groups, who can face double discrimination and disadvantage. Advocates who share an identity with the communities to which they provide advocacy services can recognise the issues and cut through layers of distrust more readily. This can involve a shared identity of ethnicity, faith, disability, age, gender or sexual orientation. Whatever the characteristic(s), arguably it is the shared experience of disadvantage, marginalisation or oppression which makes these advocacy partnerships effective.

'Hard to reach, easy to ignore'

Despite the clear importance of protecting the rights of marginalised groups, our research found wide variation in uptake of IMHA: only between 20 and 55 per cent of the total number of qualifying patients were accessing IMHA services. Furthermore, we identified five groups of qualifying patients who were particularly underserved by IMHA services, as well as those on CTOs and people placed outside their area of residence. These were people from BAME communities; people with learning difficulties; older people with dementia; people who have hearing impairments or are deaf; and children and young people under

---

4   Chapter 3 refers to some of the key critiques relevant to gendered assumptions and treatment in mental health.

5   See Andrew Solomon (2012) for an exploration of identity and difference and associated discrimination and disadvantage.

the age of 18. Indeed, a consistent theme was that people who may require IMHA support the most were least likely to access the service: 'hard to reach, easy to ignore' (Newbigging et al. 2012a, p.70). The reasons that qualifying patients gave for not accessing IMHA services included not knowing the service existed, not understanding the purpose of IMHA or assumptions about the consequences of using an IMHA. This raises questions about the commissioning, design and provision of IMHA services, including the assumptions about power, and the involvement of diverse service users so that the services live up to the aspiration of protecting rights and empowerment in its fullest sense.

People from BAME communities

Advocacy has been repeatedly identified as needed in major reports for people from BAME communities to address inequities in relation to the mental health system and wider disadvantage (Centre for Social Justice 2011; Department of Health 2005a; Keating *et al.* 2002), including inquiries into the deaths of African Caribbean men in mental health services (NSC NHS Strategic Health Authority 2003). Hakim and Pollard (2011) identified how the pace of introduction of IMHA services disadvantaged BAME advocacy, impacting on access to IMHA by people from BAME communities. This was confirmed by our research, which found evidence of significant unmet need and evidence of variation in uptake of IMHA services by people from BAME communities, raising questions about the commissioning and organisation of IMHA services for qualifying patients from these communities.

In our study, service users from BAME communities identified that their assessment of whether the organisation providing IMHA services had an understanding of the experience of marginalisation of minority ethnic communities in British society and in mental health services could influence their uptake of IMHA services. A shared understanding of the historical and contemporaneous context was also identified as an important feature of their approach by BAME advocates:

I'm not saying 'I'm Black so I understand what you're facing' and my colleague doesn't because she's not Black, that's not the way. But I think the other part of it is historically the understanding of what has been, how people have been treated in the past, how it affects people, how medication can be over-used, the side effects of that to people, how it's disabling in certain things. (BAME advocate quoted in Newbigging *et al.* 2012a, p.156)

An overly narrow emphasis on rights under the MH Act may be seen as relatively ineffective if the wider social disadvantage of BAME communities is not addressed (Centre for Social Justice 2011). Furthermore, studies have highlighted the importance of different models of advocacy to meet culturally diverse needs, including approaches that are much more embedded within communities and concerned with interdependence, with families for instance, than the defined model of independence embodied in IMHA (Mir and Nocon 2002; Rai-Atkins *et al.* 2002).

An individual's assessment not only of the capacity of an IMHA service to respond appropriately, but also that of mental health professionals, can play an important role in determining whether or not an approach will be made or a service accepted. In the following instance, an African Caribbean woman was asked whether or not her keyworker would help her access the IMHA service:

I don't trust… I don't trust her enough for that. No, I don't… I've known my keyworker for nearly twenty years, I don't trust her enough for that. I would ask someone like…do you know the African girl in the office, I'd ask her. (Non-IMHA user quoted in Newbigging *et al.* 2012a, p.156)

Some service users highlighted the importance of being clear on the IMHA's stance in relation to the mental health system, because of experiences of coercive mental health services:

You can always tell which side of the fence they're on… I can. So if this Advocacy came to see me and they seem to be leaning towards the side of the mental health team then I probably wouldn't get involved with them because you can be treated in the community, you don't need to be locked up to be treated. (IMHA partner, African Caribbean man, quoted in Newbigging *et al.* 2012a, p.157)

While it was not clear from our study whether a shared ethnic identity with the IMHA would have helped or not, an earlier study of mental health advocacy for African and African Caribbean men indicated that this was important, particularly in determining understanding of, access to and the nature of advocacy provision (Newbigging *et al.* 2007). On the other hand, sharing an ethnic identity may raise concerns for service users about confidentiality, both in relation to the service user's own community and also that of the mental health professionals:

I know from my community they have mental health issues, sometimes I see them on the ward. When they speak I know that they are from my type of community and I know that they need that service. As soon as they see me they recognise me, we recognise each other, but because we are from the same community they say 'oh, I'm fine, I don't need this service'. (IMHA, BAME advocacy organisation, quoted in Newbigging *et al.* 2012a, p.158)

The specific needs of people from BAME communities in relation to IMHA services was most often construed by IMHA providers in terms of language issues, highlighting access to interpreters as critical. This is clearly important, and if they were not readily available other patients may be expected to interpret. Arguably, this reflects a one-dimensional view of disempowerment in terms of Lukes' (2005) conceptualisation of power, and it is clear from this analysis that the issues regarding access and appropriate provision are much more profound than language. BAME advocacy providers, some of which were providing IMHA services in our study, provided a more nuanced account of the needs and advocacy for people from BAME communities. This included consideration of cultural issues, for example in relation to diet, spirituality and historical context, as discussed above and fundamental differences in conceptions of distress and advocacy. Locating advocacy services within wider community organisations was seen as having wider benefits than solely to the individual as raising awareness of mental health issues, but conversely locating BAME advocates within mainstream advocacy services also brought benefits 'because it makes them [other advocates] understand how mental health is different, perceived differently by the Asian community, and about what depression is' (BAME advocate quoted in Newbigging *et al.* 2012a, p.158).

When the issue of access for patients from BAME communities was raised with IMHA services in our study, the majority stated that anyone could access their services and that services were person centred and met the individual needs of service users. Overall, though, we found limited awareness across the mainstream IMHA providers and commissioners as to the specific needs of local BAME communities and few efforts appeared to have been made to establish these. For example, we did not find any evidence that data from the Count Me In census (CQC 2011) had been considered, or that consultation with specific community groups had taken place. The conclusion from this and previous research (Newbigging *et al.* 2007; Rai-Atkins *et al.* 2002) is that mainstream advocacy organisations may not be attractive to, or have the skills and knowledge within the staff team to provide culturally competent services for, qualifying patients from BAME communities.

People with learning difficulties

Any service that relies on patients understanding enough to request services is inherently discriminating to those who lack capacity in various aspects of their life. People with learning difficulties have struggled to receive appropriate mental health services with mental health professionals sometimes lacking the appropriate skills (Gregory *et al.* 2003). In contrast, learning disability services are likely to be more aware of capacity issues and of advocacy, reflecting the influence of normalisation and a tradition of citizen advocacy and self-advocacy. Thus people with learning difficulties who qualify for IMHA services may find it difficult to access them if they are reliant on mental health service professionals for access, but may be at an advantage if supported by learning disability services.

The lack of collaboration between mental health and learning disability services may be replicated in the organisation and delivery of advocacy services. In one of our research sites, we came across an advocacy organisation that had recently formed two organisations: one providing advocacy services for people experiencing mental health problems and the other providing independent advocacy to vulnerable people including people with learning difficulties and older people. However, only the former service was commissioned to provide IMHA services but was not providing IMHA services to any qualifying patients with learning difficulties, thus creating a gap in provision. The other service then found itself in a difficult position: understanding the specific needs of people with learning difficulties but not having any advocates qualified as IMHAs nor being commissioned to provide this service. In another site, the commissioners developed two separate service specifications – one for instructed and one for non-instructed advocacy services – and included the IMHA provision in the specification for instructed advocacy. This immediately created a gap in provision for people who qualified for IMHA services but lacked the capacity to instruct an advocate. In contrast, an IMHA manager in another area had experience of working with people with learning difficulties and it was evident that this service was taking active steps to ensure access and that people's needs were actively considered in service provision.

Facilitating access to IMHA services for people with learning difficulties requires detailed attention overall to communication and providing information in appropriate formats. We identified notable examples of good practice:

The majority of them [IMHAs] who have been with us for more than 12 months have been on inclusive communication training so there's myself and another Advocate who are trained in the use of talking mats and then there's myself and another Advocate who are trained in Makaton Sign Language and there's a third Advocate who's trained in British Sign

Language, so between us we do have these skills within the service. (IMHA manager quoted in Newbigging *et al.* 2012a, p.161)

As with older people, there may be an issue for people with learning difficulties who lack capacity, in relation to access to non-instructed advocacy.

Older adults

Older adults detained under the MH Act may be particularly vulnerable and, as a higher proportion may lack the capacity to instruct an advocate, as a consequence of dementia. There may also be issues in relation to safeguarding as older people can be vulnerable to abuse and exploitation. Use of IMHA services for older people was identified by our research as a major gap in provision. Given that IMHA services have developed from generic mental health advocacy, provision of non-instructed advocacy is generally a less familiar way of working. Thus, in our study, some older adults qualifying for IMHA services without the capacity to instruct an IMHA were missing out on this service:

> I think that's a historical thing that up until the IMHA Service came in we weren't able to work with those people, we weren't funded to work with those people because we had to work with people that could instruct us and tell us what they want and quite often the older adults who were detained especially aren't able to do that, so that's been again quite a struggle... I'm well aware that there are people there that aren't being referred to us, especially for the Older Adults Units. (Advocacy manager quoted in Newbigging *et al.* 2012a, p.153)

As noted in Chapter 6, provision of advocacy in general for people with dementia is patchy (Dementia Advocacy Network 2013) and we found few IMHA providers who had developed their provision specifically for older people with dementia. Overall, the uptake of IMHA services on wards for older adults was relatively low, which was in part attributed to close involvement of family members and a reluctance by the older people to seek external help. However, as IMHAs may not be regular visitors to such wards, or may be more reluctant to use non-instructed advocacy, older people may be being disadvantaged. Our findings indicate that either staff need to routinely refer all qualifying patients and/or IMHA services need to visit older people's wards and be ready to provide non-instructed advocacy. Engaging with families and carers, as in other contexts, could increase the uptake of IMHA services.

People with physical and/or sensory impairment

For people with physical and sensory impairments, the main issue identified by our study was securing appropriate provision for hearing impaired and Deaf people, particularly people who were born deaf or became deaf in early childhood. Deaf people are a linguistic minority and, in 2003, British Sign Language (BSL) was recognized as a language in its own right (National Mental Health Development Unit 2011).

Deaf people have struggled for access and equality for many years and have limited access to mainstream services. Sometimes that is because they are not aware the service exists, but it is often because the service is not delivered through BSL interpreters, and the staff have no understanding of the needs of Deaf people (Essery 2014). In relation to mental health, Information from Sign Health indicates that 40% of Deaf people will suffer from some form of mental illness once in their lifetime, compared to 25% of hearing people and there are high levels of unmet need, most likely reflecting the barriers faced by Deaf people in accessing adequate mental health assessments and services at all levels (Sign and Mental Health Foundation, undated). Deaf people are over-represented in forensic services and a number of specialist units exist in England (Sign and Mental Health Foundation, undated).

In our study, communication was identified as essential in facilitating access to IMHAs but cultural competence was also necessary. Access to IMHAs who can sign was identified as being more effective than a hearing advocate with a BSL interpreter, both in terms of establishing rapport with the service user and the cost. However, as with people from BAME communities, an understanding of, or identity within the Deaf culture was also highlighted. A ward manager on a specialist Deaf unit commented that for some people, an unqualified deaf advocate would be preferred to a hearing IMHA:

> A deaf person won't... you know especially someone that's mentally ill responding to their own or whatever, so a hearing person coming in who will then need to use an interpreter, that would cause a barrier straight away with the patient, so I would imagine that the pick-up would be poor. (Ward Manager quoted in Newbigging et al. 2012a, p.162)

Just as in the case of BAME advocacy organizations, it was found to be the case that some specialist Deaf advocates were from advocacy organizations that were not funded specifically to provide IMHA services but they did so out of concern for unmet need. Figure 10.1 provides an example of such a service.

BOX 10.1 SIGNHEALTH

SignHealth offers a wide variety of support to deaf people with health issues and campaigns for equality and improved access to health services for deaf people. Due to government cuts, social services have been closing services for deaf people. Therefore community advocacy is becoming more and more important. The majority of SignHealth advocates are deaf themselves, because deaf advocates are better able to empathise and understand deaf people's needs. They can also communicate fluently in British Sign Language on a one-to-one basis (without the need for an interpreter). It is difficult for a hearing person to attend a BSL course to learn the language as deaf people have a particular grassroots way of using the language that is not easily learnt by a hearing person.

SignHealth Advocacy supports deaf people to fight these inequalities, but statutory funding is only available for IMHA and IMCA. The Care Act 2014 makes provision for the use of advocacy to support people who lack capacity in the community. Those deaf people who require support but do not fall under any of these statutory categories struggle to attract funding for advocacy.

(Source: Sign Health, Frank Essery, Senior Advocate, IMHA and IMCA)

Children and young people

Children and young people detained under the MH Act 1983 are eligible for IMHA services, irrespective of age, and in addition if they are under 18 years and their clinician is considering ECT. They are at risk of not receiving appropriate care and, prior to amendments of the MH Act 2007, may have been placed in unsafe and inappropriate adult settings where they might experience physical or sexual abuse (Children's Commissioner for England 2007). Further, they may face instability and upheaval associated with having been in care (Chase 2008) or being placed in a specialist unit some distance away from their family. Access to independent advocacy has been identified as an important safeguard (11 Million and Young Minds 2008; Street *et al.* 2012). However, in terms of availability, independence and accessibility, children and young people's access to advocacy has been described as a 'postcode lottery' with particular gaps in meeting the needs of the most vulnerable young people, including those with mental health problems (Brady 2011). Wood and Selwyn (2013) arrived at similar conclusions when they set out to examine the characteristics of looked after young people using independent advocacy services across the country.

In our study few children and young people were accessing IMHA services, and there were differences between areas in the extent to which areas were commissioning specific provision for children and young people. In some parts of the country we found dedicated IMHA services for children and young people and, in two instances, this was provided separately from the adult service, whilst in one it was part of the same service. One national children's service commissioned to provide IMHA reported no uptake so far, and other IMHA providers had had very few referrals of children and young people under 16. Similar patchiness in provision of advocacy services for children and young people making complaints about mental health services was noted by Street et al. (2012) in a study for the Children's Commissioner for England. They found that not all CAMHS in-patient units had advocacy services, and this lack of independent support affected children and young people's ability to make a complaint.

There are a number of barriers that children and young people may face in accessing IMHA services. From a scoping exercise to map general advocacy provision for children and young people in England, Brady (2011) identified the following barriers that children and young people can face in accessing advocacy services, which are particularly relevant to accessing IMHA provision:

- lack of knowledge about advocacy

- physical barriers, such as staffing levels and the type of telephone used by the service provider

- communication barriers, particularly for younger children or those less able to articulate their views

- language barriers for children and young people whose first language isn't English

- confidentiality barriers and the dilemma between safeguarding rights and protecting children

- emotional barriers, reflecting young people's lack of confidence in themselves.

Other studies have found that children and young people generally do not have much awareness of advocacy and its availability (Street *et al.* 2012).

The power differential that exists in relation to age may also serve as a barrier in settings where all staff will be adults. Thus, the profile and visibility (in order to build up familiarity and trust in the advocacy service) will go some way to addressing these issues. Children and young people will require a different style of advocacy, including specially designed leaflets and a resource pack to promote self-advocacy.[6]

LGBT people

Although not specifically highlighted in our study, it was notable that IMHA services were less likely to record sexual orientation and therefore it was hard to evaluate the extent to which IMHA services were meeting the needs of people from LGBT groups. No specific provision for LGBT was identified in any of the case study sites, nor was this raised by any of the participants, although the sample did include people who identified as gay or bisexual. One of the IMHA services, where we undertook a shadow visit, had secured funding to work with LGBT people experiencing mental health difficulties, primarily in the community but also in hospital, and worked with an IMHA colleague to meet the needs of LGBT service users who were detained. As noted earlier, the co-location of mental health advocacy within an LGBT service was highly valued by service users (PACE 2008), suggesting that similar issues relating to service identity could facilitate access.

Responses to diversity

The findings discussed above challenge the assumption in the sector that because IMHA services are 'person centred' they are meeting the needs of the diverse populations they serve.

6   See for example Maze Advocacy in Somerset. Resources available at
     http://mazeadvocacy.net (accessed on 24 January 2015).

Furthermore, there is little evidence of strategic planning to address specific needs in the commissioning and design of IMHA services. A range of potential remedies to address the inequities in provision is available: these include legal and practical remedies, with implications for commissioning of IMHA services; the operation of IMHA services; and the profile and skills of IMHAs.

Legal remedies

Framing mental health within a human and civil rights discourse has the potential to expose the injustice done to various groups as well as providing recourse through the courts, although the effectiveness of such measures is debatable. In an era of new medicalism, as discussed in Chapter 4, there is a tendency for the courts to uphold decisions made on medical grounds (Richardson 2008). Although the law provides safeguards to protect rights, earlier discussion illustrates how its implementation may disadvantage particular groups. Overall, there has been scant research in this area, and that which exists has tended to focus on ethnicity, reflecting the profile of African Caribbean groups in relation to compulsion under the MH Act. However, a retrospective analysis of appeals found that people identified as Black Caribbean or White Irish were much more likely to appeal than those identified as White British (Nilforooshan, Amin and Warner 2009). Despite high rates of appeal overall, the success of such appeals was low. This raises some interesting questions about the purpose and conduct of appeals and may also indicate greater dissatisfaction with treatment and care amongst these groups.

The Equality Act 2010 provides the legal framework for ensuring that specific groups of people are not disadvantaged and makes it unlawful to discriminate (directly or indirectly) against a person on the basis of a protected characteristic or combination of protected characteristics. There are nine protected characteristics under the equality legislation: age; disability; gender reassignment; marriage and civil partnership; maternity and pregnancy; race; religion and belief; sex; and sexual orientation. Disability includes mental impairment that has a substantial and long-term adverse effect on the person's ability to carry out normal day-to-day activities. The Equality Duty applies to most public services, and this will include voluntary sector services, commissioned to provide advocacy. The Equality Duty has three aims:

- to eliminate unlawful harassment and discrimination

- to advance equality of opportunity for people with protected characteristics between people who share a protected characteristic and people who do not share it

- to foster good relations between people who share a protected characteristic and people who do not share it.

(Government Equalities Office 2012, p.3)

In addition, the Equality Act requires public sector organisations to make reasonable adjustments so that people with protected characteristics get the same level of services as people without. In terms of IMHA provision, not providing an interpreter or information in an accessible format would contravene this requirement. Advocacy, itself, can also be thought of as a reasonable adjustment (NDTi 2012) and strengthens the argument for IMHA to be provided on an opt-out rather than an opt-in basis (House of Commons 2013). A review of advocacy in social care for protected groups undertaken by the Equality and Human Rights Commission (2010) did not point to further legislative measures but concluded that outreach and collaborative working, including creating a single point of access, would improve advocacy for these groups. Undertaking an equality analysis as part of the commissioning process and in designing services will help determine local solutions to ensure that the advocacy needs of the whole population, including groups with protected characteristics, are met. This will necessarily require engagement with diverse groups in order to consider particular needs and ways of addressing any potential disadvantage, such as those identified in the earlier discussion.

Policy remedies

The policy framework for health and social care in general, and mental health in particular, can also provide a steer for commissioners, mental health services and IMHA services as to the nature of inequities people face, and support action to address these. Under the Labour administration, there was a clear intent to address inequities in relation to mental health, and the early to mid-twenty-first century saw several policy documents that described the nature of these inequities and outlined action to address them. Of particular note was Delivering Race Equality (DRE) (Department of Health 2005b) that aimed to address the position of people from BAME communities in respect of mental health in response to an inquiry into the death of David (Rocky) Bennett. It identified three key actions to address this:

1. better, more responsive services, which includes advocacy

2. better engagement of services with BAME communities

3. better information.

This was supported by investment in a programme of activity under the auspices of the NIMHE to support the implementation of the DRE policy objectives. Alongside DRE, NIMHE also developed policy and invested in implementation support in respect of women (Department of Health 2003), older adults and children and young people. Initiatives to address the stigma and marginalisation of people with mental health problems were also introduced (Wilson 2009). These initiatives were not formally evaluated but were considered to have led to shifts in practice and attitudes through acknowledging the need to promote equality and reduce inequities (Newbigging et al. 2010; Wilson 2009).

Although health inequities remain on the agenda with the work of Michael Marmot,[7] the translation of this into

---

7   See for example the Institute of Health Equity. Available at: www.instituteofhealthequity.org (accessed on 25 January 2015).

specific actions in relation to mental health is, as yet, unclear. The focus on specific characteristics has been lost since 2010, although current mental health policy devotes a whole chapter to promoting equalities in mental health, locating this within the context of the Equality Act. The lack of focus has drawn attention elsewhere, with Craig (2013) commenting on the invisibilising of race within current policy. Equally, proponents of mainstreaming in relation to gender equity have pointed to the importance of targeted action to ensure equity objectives are met alongside actions to mainstream gender within all policies (Newbigging *et al.* 2010; Ravindran and Kelkar-Khambete 2008). In the absence of the latter, there is scope for local discretion and a risk that a technocratic approach to equity will prevail.

Practical remedies

Within these legal and policy frameworks that promote equality, commissioners and providers have many opportunities to progress this agenda, and failure to do so points to deep-seated resistance indicative of Lukes' third dimension of power.

COMMISSIONING FOR EQUITY IN IMHA SERVICES

In Chapter 12, we consider commissioning IMHA services in detail and make it clear that good commissioning is underpinned by co-production with people who use services, carers and families, and communities. Box 10.2 provides an overview of the key steps commissioners can take to ensure the equitable provision of IMHA services.

BOX 10.2 MEASURES FOR COMMISSIONERS TO ENSURE EQUITY IN RESPECT OF IMHA

The measures are:

- engage service users, carers, advocates and communities in the commissioning process

- design services grounded in identified need and agreed outcomes, and reflecting local demography

- adopt a strategic approach to the development of mental health advocacy, based on a holistic approach to empowerment

- ensure equality of access to high-quality and effective mental health advocacy through investment in the building capacity of mainstream advocacy organisations and community organisations

- understand and value diverse ways of providing mental health advocacy, including commissioning community and micro-organisations to provide IMHA services

- provide sustainable funding for advocacy to support open access to IMHA services

- work with CCGs in commissioning mental health services that ensure measures are in place to promote and support access to IMHA services for all

- monitor and review access to, uptake of and experience of IMHA services for diverse groups of people subject to compulsion.

(Source: Adapted from Newbigging et al. 2008)

The foundation for commissioning IMHA services is engagement with people who have experience of compulsion from different communities. This is likely to be a challenging task as a consequence of the stigma associated with detention, the distressing nature of the experience and the circumstances surrounding it. Gathering relevant information about the profile of people subject to compulsion, however, is a critical step, and historically, as we found in our study, the NHS has been poor at doing this. This will necessarily involve both considering data on detentions by different groups (currently only available on age, race and gender) alongside engagement with people from diverse communities to build a nuanced picture of the barriers and facilitators to access and use of IMHA services. The experience from DRE of developing community engagement methods to understand the perspectives of particular communities illustrates the importance of working with community members and investing in community organisations to understand the real-life complexities of engagement with the mental health system (Wilson 2009). Another approach being pioneered by Essex County Council is the use of ethnographic research approaches to develop a holistic appreciation of people's lives:

> Traditionally we will have run focus groups, done surveys, we will have asked people directly what they think. Ethnography is about getting right underneath the skin of people's real life stories. What are their insights? What innovations have they got? Might they even be part of the solution to the problem? We're really interested in pursuing the whole process of commissioning in a much more transparent, much more open way. (Dave Hill, Executive Director for People Commissioning)[8]

Both these approaches would have benefits to communities and to the commissioning of wider mental health and wider services than IMHA.

---

8   Source: Essex County Council, http://essexpartnership.org/content/ ethnographic-research (accessed on 25 January 2014).

This information should inform a Joint Strategic Needs Assessment (JSNA), which local authorities are required under the legislation to produce about their local area and commissioning decisions about how to provide effective IMHA services that achieve the outcomes that people want. There are three key decisions facing commissioners and their partners, the outcome of which will influence the access to and uptake of IMHA services. First, commissioners need to decide on the scope of the service model in terms of its purpose and the people that it will be designed to serve. Issues relating to purpose are explored in Chapter 12, but in essence the key question is to what extent the service will be focused on the requirements of the MH Act (i.e. negative rights) and to what extent the service will support the wider empowerment of people subject to the Act (i.e. positive rights). We refer to this as the protection–empowerment debate.

Second, commissioners need to decide whether or not to adopt a policy of open access given the difficulties regarding access that we have discussed earlier. Open access means that there is a proactive approach so that people have to opt out rather than opt in to use IMHA services. This was recommended in our original research, reinforced by the recent scrutiny of the Mental Health Act (House of Commons 2013)[9]. This will have funding implications that are, as yet, untested. Adopting an open access policy also means that the IMHA service needs to be funded for advocates to have the time to be available on a ward so that detained patients can have the opportunity to meet an IMHA to help them decide whether it's for them or not.

Third, commissioners need to decide on what are the best organisational arrangements to ensure that the advocacy needs of all qualifying patients are met. There is a general trend for local authorities to reduce the transaction costs of managing multiple contracts by going for large organisations that can fulfil a number of functions. The landscape of advocacy provision, as was discussed in Chapter 7, is increasingly dominated by organisations

---

9   Although not supported in the response from the Department of Health, who indicated the need for primary legislation to achieve this (Department of Health 2013).

that cover a region or the whole country, and which provide a range of different types of advocacy. It is understood that smaller organisations often fare poorly in bidding processes because they lack the infrastructure to respond quickly to tendering processes, which, therefore, need to be proportionate to encourage such organisations to bid (Carr 2014). However, the issues are more complex, and the relative merits of mainstream organisations versus smaller community-led organisations are summarised in Table 10.1. This typology is derived from a national survey of advocacy organisations (Newbigging *et al.* 2007), and given the recent developments in the landscape of provision (see Chapter 7) it may be somewhat dated but does provide a framework for commissioners to reflect on the relationship between the type of organisational model and capacity to meet the diverse needs of the local population. As Table 10.1 illustrates, there is a potential trade-off between developed expertise and capacity around independent professional advocacy, as per IMHA, and sensitivity to the specific needs of particular groups, including well-established networks, forms of collective advocacy and provision of models of advocacy, other than independent professional advocacy.

TABLE 10.1 TYPOLOGY OF DIFFERENT ARRANGEMENTS FOR THE PROVISION OF ADVOCACY SERVICES

Type of organisation	Description	Advantages	Disadvantages
Advocacy focused.	Service model tends to be based on independent professional advocacy with collective and peer advocacy provided less frequently than individual casework.	Brings together different forms of statutory advocacy and, therefore, likely to have specialist knowledge of advocacy provision. Organisational size confers advantages in terms of training and reducing transactional costs for commissioners.	May have arrangements in place to ensure sensitivity to a wide range of needs, e.g. employing staff with specific skills, partnership arrangements with community organisations, but studies indicate this is uncommon. Tendency to adopt a uniform model that may not be sensitive to the local context.
Specialist advocacy focused on people with specific needs, e.g. children and young people, people with learning disabilities, deaf people, women.	Provides a range of advocacy for specific client groups, and may include peer advocacy, citizen advocacy and collective advocacy.	Organisations provide different forms of advocacy and advocates likely to have lived experience. Have detailed knowledge of the issues faced by the client group.	Organisations vary as to whether or not they provide IMHA services. May be viewed by commissioners as being too narrow and specialist.

Community organisations, e.g. African and Caribbean mental health services, BAME organisations.	Range of organisational arrangements from community organisations constituted around a single ethnic group providing general welfare support and advice to culturally specific and sensitive services focused on mental health to specific communities, typically as an alternative to the mainstream NHS.	Sensitised to the cultural and other issues facing the particular group. Often involved in collective advocacy on behalf of the specific client group in relation to broader civil rights.	Size may disadvantage them in the tendering process.
		All staff engaged in advocacy for the community as part of their role. Able to provide culturally sensitive advocacy, encompassing a conception of community advocacy in contrast to individual advocacy. Collective advocacy on behalf of communities in the gaps in provision and negative experiences of engagement with mental health services. Local ownership and accountability.	For general community organisations, the mission is not always articulated as advocacy but their work has clear advocacy strands. Community organisations focused on mental health may be small and disadvantaged in the tendering process.

EQUITABLE IMHA SERVICES

The capacity of IMHA services to respond to diverse needs will reflect the type of organisation and model of advocacy, as discussed above. Critical to effective IMHA services is the involvement of people with experiences of compulsion in the design and monitoring of those services. Surprisingly, we found this to be rare, possibly because some of the advocates had service user experience, but this does not negate having a range of measures in place to ensure that people from different groups and with different experiences of compulsion are well represented in the management of the IMHA service.

For IMHA services to ensure that people subject to compulsion are not being disadvantaged in accessing IMHA services, gathering information on their characteristics is an essential first step. This requires a comparison being made between the characteristics of people being detained under the MH Act and those accessing the IMHA service. The quality of information kept is generally poor, making such comparisons unlikely, with CQC reports consistently noting that the gender and ethnicity of people subject to the MH Act is not being monitored (CQC 2013). This suggests that other characteristics are not being considered for routine monitoring by NHS Trusts, for example in relation to sexual orientation or faith, although these may be considered during CQC visits.

Although IMHA services may routinely collect information on age, sex and race, our study identified reluctance on the part of IMHA services to ask about sexual orientation, and therefore information relating to all protected characteristics will be incomplete. This is consistent with a more comprehensive survey of advocacy for people with protected characteristics (Equality and Human Rights Commission 2010). There is a risk that using administrative categories can lead to homogenisation, for example of BAME and LGBT people, and stereotyping (Carr 2014). Furthermore, the way in which protected characteristics intersect in the context of the MH Act is poorly understood, potentially negating the reality that people have complex identities leading to a reductionist approach, which compounds discrimination and inequalities. IMHA services, along with commissioners, therefore need to understand the profile of people subject to compulsion in their area and the nature of the barriers to accessing and using IMHA services as well as the social context for their distress, but be alert to the risks of coming to false conclusions. For example, an easy assumption to make would be that because the IMHA workforce is predominantly female, the advocacy needs of women are being appropriately met. However, a predominance of female staff does not guarantee the gender sensitivity of IMHA services, and in particular the gendered nature of abuse and the re-traumatisation potential through the use of of compulsory measures needs to be understood.

Addressing the barriers to unequal access requires more than providing interpretation services and information in different formats. It also means services becoming culturally competent and, if the relevant skills, knowledge and sensitivities are not available in-house, forging relationships with specialist and/or community organisations. Some people, but by no means everybody, appreciate having access to advocates who understand their culture and experience of oppression and disadvantage, and who speak the same language. This is often not possible to achieve, however, within small advocacy teams with limited resources, but services can work more closely with specialist and community organisations who do have this understanding and expertise. If the IMHA service is provided by a mainstream advocacy service, they should be working in partnership with community organisations learning from them and upskilling them, if needed, to develop the skills to provide IMHA services. This would include training and support as well as shadowing, and clearly the benefits would be mutual, with mainstream advocacy organisations developing their understanding and practice in relation to these groups (see for example Westminster Advocacy Service for Senior Residents and Dementia Advocacy Network 2009). Such partnerships support outreach and the development of innovative approaches. Below are some key messages for IMHA providers to improve equality of access to IMHA services:

- As a service with a public function, IMHA is subject to a general equality duty under the Equality Act 2010.

- To develop a targeted and effective service, IMHA providers must understand the needs of the local population and especially the demographic profile of people being treated under the Mental Health Act.

- To enable the monitoring of differences in IMHA uptake it is important that the equality data of people who use these services is consistently recorded.

- Cooperating with community organisations that already deliver support and/or advocacy to particular groups is the key to meeting diverse needs.

- An equitable service must organise interpretation services, and also consider the communication styles and formats which are easiest and best for specific groups of service users.

- An advocate's identity, sensitivity and knowledge of a specific group are all crucial when it comes to gaining the trust of service users.

- Opening up IMHA to diverse communities is not just a question of service delivery but is also about adopting a principled approach that mirrors equality concerns.

(Source: SCIE/UClan 2015)[10]

Conclusions

While IMHA services that adopt an approach that is person centred will go some way to meeting individual needs, in this chapter we have argued, with reference to Lukes' (2005) conceptualisation of three levels of power, that a more

---

10   See the Useful Resources section.

sophisticated understanding of powerlessness and oppression is needed for independent advocacy services to be truly effective and equitable. Not only is it important that IMHA services take active steps through, for instance, ensuring that operational and staffing policies help them respond to the diverse needs of the qualifying population they serve, commissioners also need to address equality issues in local provision, and we expand upon this more in Chapter 12. It is clear from our own user experience, as well as the evidence from research, that taking a one- or even two-dimensional view of power falls short, and will not address the deep-rooted and historical oppressions that are manifest in the fabric of the mental health system. That said, there is much that local IMHA services together with commissioners can do to address barriers to accessing IMHA, in partnership with service users and local communities.

Responding positively to the issues and barriers identified in this chapter needs to be at three main levels: (1) through legislation framing mental health within a human and civil rights framework and promoting equality of opportunity; (2) through commissioning practices that promote equality; and (3) through IMHA services whose practices and staff are sensitive to and understand the different barriers particular groups face in accessing services and their wider historical and social context.

REFLECTIVE EXERCISES

1. With reference to the issues discussed in this chapter, list the most common issues leading to inequities in access to effective IMHA services and the groups most affected.

2. Consider the strategies that IMHA services can use to become more aware of the barriers some groups, for example young people or people from BAME communities, face in accessing appropriate IMHA services, and how they might address these within existing resources. How can advocacy services avoid tick box approaches?

3. Who else needs to ensure that access to effective and appropriate IMHA services is accessible to all? Outline the responsibilities of commissioners and policy makers, for example.

4. Identify the key elements of an equitable IMHA service including the staffing and operational policies that would need to be in place. Draft a model operational policy for an IMHA service that aims to address inequity in access to its service.

Chapter 11

RELATIONSHIPS WITH
SERVICE PROVIDERS

Introduction

This chapter explores the relationship between mental health service staff and advocacy services, and the importance of constructive relations for effective advocacy. We present a descriptive matrix of the different forms such relationships might our take, derived from the findings of our study (McKeown *et al.* 2014; Newbigging *et al.* 2012). We begin by addressing the claims for an advocacy role on the part of mental health service staff themselves, and how these, despite well-meaning intentions, can not replace truly independent advocacy. Furthermore, we suggest that it is a naive view of advocacy and confusion over who can take on an advocacy role in this provider context that contributes to strained working relationships and negative views about independent advocates.

In our study of IMHA, we elicited the views of mental health staff, managers, commissioners, practising advocates and service users. The findings reinforce other research and commentary that have drawn attention to certain practical and conceptual tensions between the advocates and mental health service provider staff (Carver and Morrison 2005; McKeown *et al.* 2002). Notably, there was variable appreciation for, or understanding of, the very idea of independent advocacy amongst mental health staff. This confusion extended to uncertainties regarding the limitations of staff's assumptions of an advocacy role or empowerment philosophy. Perhaps more importantly, difficulties were evident in contemplation of the contribution of mental health staff in supporting the work of independent advocates.

Whilst the presence of staff with progressive values and an affinity for advocacy is desirable, these alone are insufficient for optimal working relations unless they also possess sufficient understanding of the importance of independence. Conclusions are drawn concerning healthy and constructive relations and how to best achieve them – seeking to optimise circumstances whereby staff such as nurses and social workers (usually in the role of AMHP) can be supported to both appreciate the value of advocacy and to understand it fully.

Institutional support for advocacy

There are a number of expectations for mental health services and their personnel to support the provision of advocacy, and some of these are legally obligated. These are set out in detail in the revised MH Act Code of Practice (Department of Health 2015). Commissioning arrangements have provided for various communication and feedback processes to be built into contracts; however, most liaison is fairly informal and occurs between advocates and hospital ward staff. The quality of this communication can vary greatly, ranging from welcoming teams who keep the advocate informed of changes for qualifying patients, to failures to pass on key information, extend invitations to meetings or even to be civil in routine interactions. In this regard, arrangements for CPA or case review meetings can represent an indicative test of working relationships. Nursing staff are obliged to support advocates' legal rights to access case records with permission of qualifying patients. Practical assistance for advocacy includes identifying and protecting space on the ward for advocates to meet with qualifying patients, and ensuring their safety via communicating simple information about perceived risks in advance of meetings. In some settings advocates are issued personal alarms or access personal safety training.

Services also have a role in promoting advocacy, including ensuring that qualifying patients and staff know the appropriate channels for contacting the advocacy service providing IMHAs, and that staff have a working understanding of advocacy sufficient to make appropriate referrals and meet their statutory duties. Our study found that despite extant programmes of training and induction aimed at clinical staff, basic comprehension can be lacking, and in some instances available training is cursory or inadequate.

The advocacy role of professionals

For some time, various professional disciplines have claimed to operate an advocacy role in health or social care settings, most notably nurses and social workers. This speaks to the value in professional staff considering their role in challenging the points of view and perspectives of colleagues, working to uphold client and patient rights, and promoting involvement and participation in care and treatment. For example, advocacy has long been recognised as central to the social work role, with effective social work advocacy practice being fundamental to promoting individual rights and social justice (Dalrymple and Boylan 2013). These authors date the timeline for advocacy within social work back to the early 1800s, asserting that health and social work professionals have a 'crucial role to play in promoting rights, participation and service user involvement' (2013, p.x) alongside independent advocacy. Many international nursing regulatory frameworks also promote advocacy as part of the expected nursing role, and this is often dated to the enactment of the United Nations Declaration on the Rights of Disabled People in 1975 (Jugessur and Iles 2009). This was taken up by the United Kingdom Central Council for nursing in 1996. In the UK the Nursing and Midwifery Council (2004) obligates nurses to 'promote the interests of patients and clients' and, similarly, social workers are urged to be responsible for acting as advocates for their clients (Bateman 2000).

Nelson (1988) dates nurses' interest in advocacy to Florence Nightingale and argues this has moved from simple intercession on behalf of individuals to a more sophisticated guardianship of rights and protection of client autonomy, individually and collectively. In all domains of health care, not limited to mental health, it is possible to find service users whose health condition renders them unable to exercise their autonomy or for this to be in some way restricted. Such circumstances often place nurses in a position of advocating for service users, and this has latterly been framed in terms of defending human rights (Stylianos and Kehyayan 2012, p.118). With regard to staff training, advocates can have a key role in education about rights protection (Stylianos and Kehyayan 2012, p.118); conceivably this should target service users too (Reville and Church 2012).

For professional practice disciplines such as nursing and social work, interest in the advocacy role is bound up with values and principles of caring, social justice and empowerment (Dalrymple and Boylan 2013). In the mental health context, specific papers have explored nursing advocacy in such instances as the course of processes for ensuring informed consent (Usher and Arthur 1998) and medication compliance (Happell et al. 2002). In forensic settings, which are arguably even more disempowering for service users, nurses could also claim a counter-balancing advocacy role (Holmes 2001). Critical commentators agree that this should be part of a set of professional, intellectual and political concerns which respect the rights and dignity of the most disadvantaged individuals who are subject to control and surveillance and who are least likely to have their voice heard (Bindman *et al.* 2003; Gostin 2000), but dispute whether such ideals of advocacy are actually realised by professional mental health occupations (Holmes 2001). In this sense Holmes is urging nurses to assume at least two forms of advocacy: one at the level of individual cases in the practice domain; the other with respect to raising concerns in the public sphere, for instance about abusive or neglectful aspects of institutional care regimes. In a study of mental health nursing in Australian acute in-patient environments, Cleary (2004, p.56) found that the nurses typically voiced 'a clear personal philosophy of advocacy and attempted to structure nursing interactions to promote client autonomy and informed choice'.

More often than not, a perceived nursing advocacy role is presented fairly uncritically in terms of nurses' interest in patient welfare and safety. If limitations are recognised they are often seen in terms of tensions between concerns for individual voice, allegiances to employer or colleagues, unfettered managerialism devoted to cost cutting, prevailing power imbalances or paternalistic medical dominance (Jenny 1979; Jugessur and Iles 2009; Miller, Manson and Lee 1983; Pullen 1995; Robinson 1985; Vaartio *et al.* 2006; Walsh 1985; Zomorodi and Foley 2009) and, as such, are essentially about compromised independence. For these reasons Jugessur and Iles (2009) argue for more sophisticated understandings of nurse advocacy, including attention to location within prevailing legal frameworks and more clarity regarding boundaries, so that nurses have better guidance so as not to overstep the dividing line with independent advocacy practice:

> It would be appropriate for future studies to help determine a clearly relevant model of nurse advocacy in mental health nursing and for the voice of those people who have used or are using mental health services to offer some insight into their experiences. (Jugessur and Iles 2009, p.193)

Whilst supporting independent advocacy, Bateman (1995, 2000) has been a vigorous proselytiser for health and social care professionals adopting some form of advocacy role and utilising appropriate skills to do so. This is bound up with a passionate concern with democratising the relations of health and social care service delivery. For example, Teasdale (1999, p.vii) also urges professional social welfare staff to assume an advocacy role and challenge the disempowerment of service users within contemporary services, but he also identifies risks and issues a warning to avoid becoming 'bruised and battered as a result of trying to stand up and be counted as advocates'.

Thus advocacy has been framed as a collective professional responsibility, which addresses the socio-economic determinants of health (see Hubinette *et al.* 2014) or is concerned with a more radical orientation. It can be argued that the latter has been a distinct feature of the professionalisation history of social work practice, without ever achieving dominance within the discipline (e.g. Collins 2009; Ferguson and Lavalette 2006). The Social Work Action Network (SWAN), a network of social work practitioners, academics, students and social welfare users, has recently reclaimed a professional identity as the challenger of oppression, poverty and disadvantage, promoting a model of social work thinking and practice that values both individual relationship-based interventions and collective approaches (Jones et al. 2004). Jugessur and Iles (2009) trace the introduction of advocacy as part of the role of the mental health nurse to the 1970s, associated with affinity for humanistic and ethical approaches to empowerment.

At a time when independent advocacy was fairly new in the UK, Craig (1998) highlighted the correspondence of advocacy's social justice and emancipatory roots with similar objectives amidst radical collectives of health and social care professionals. Ultimately, she depicts advocacy as a key contributor to a broader transformative mission of democratisation and humanisation within services and also extending to society at large. In this regard Bateman (2000, p.9) concurs:

> How far a society is able to tolerate and encourage advocacy is a test of that society's commitment to democracy and pluralism... Advocacy thus raises fundamental questions about the nature of a society, its constitution and its respect for individuals. The greater the furtherance of advocacy the healthier that society is.

Notwithstanding this positive framing of professionals' advocacy role, Ryles (1999) pointed out how mental health nursing's expressed affinities for an empowerment role is misconceived unless nurses can collectively develop a more politicised understanding of power relations in practice. This must crucially involve recognition of, and resistance to, the extent to which nurses themselves are subject to power exercised through the dominance of a biomedical psychiatric hegemony. Arguably, part of the way in which nursing and other groups might extricate themselves from this trap must be grounded in the activities, research and teaching of academic colleagues, perhaps in association with mental health social movements – in this regard there has been a mixed response (Cresswell and Spandler 2013).

The fact that there have been some notable nurse whistleblowing cases demonstrates at least to some extent that practitioner staff can put their own interests to one side and advocate for service users' welfare, rights and entitlements (Ahern and McDonald 2002; Jackson 2008). In our study, an independent advocacy contribution could provide for solutions in circumstances where staff lacked the necessary power or leverage to bring about change:

> Staff realise that they can be helped too by some of our legitimate criticisms and complaints to the middle management because sometimes when qualified staff make these…it goes nowhere, whereas with the advocate you know they have to…take note. (Service user quoted in McKeown *et al.* 2014a, p.403)

More critically it should be acknowledged that for professionals to be advocates 'such a worker would usually have to act outside the scope of his/her agency and work role, and/or reject rather than implement its society-mandated policies' (Wolfensberger 1977 cited in Brandon and Brandon 2000), which would clearly present major challenges both to nurses and social workers in a mental health context. In the learning disability services context, Ryan and Thomas (1980) remarked that 'the staff of our institutions would be doing both themselves and mentally handicapped people a great service if they could see themselves as part of the problem and not just the solution' (p.152). Thus, Wilson and Beresford (2000, p.567) argue that social workers (and by implication other care staff) need to consider 'their own role in the creation and perpetuation of such oppression' – working as AMHPs, for instance. Furthermore, the idea of professionals like nurses advocating for their patients is under-researched from the patients' perspective (Jugessur and Iles 2009).

(Mis)understanding the advocacy role

The principle of independence was found by our research into the quality of IMHA to be paramount for effective and authentic advocacy, and this can only be achieved if advocates are not employed by the same organisation responsible for care delivery (Barnes *et al.* 2002; Harrison and Davis 2009; Newbigging *et al.* 2012a). Importantly, this ensures that the person charged with the advocacy role is free to speak without prejudicing themselves, which, for the reasons highlighted above, can never be truly the case for staff performing advocacy. For Teasdale (1999), many of the situations best served by professionals assuming an advocacy role involve efforts to clarify what a person's wishes are. However, the need for independent advocacy is most obviously made when these wishes are in conflict with what staff and service providers consider is reasonable and possibly also within the boundaries of available resources for which staff act as gatekeepers.

Findings from our IMHA study suggest that mutual understanding of roles is pivotal in predicting better-quality relationships between mental health staff and advocates: 'Each understanding a bit more of each other's service and you know them [IMHAs] understanding a bit more of what constraints we're under... So it's just that bit more understanding on both parts' (ward manager, acute ward, quoted in Newbigging *et al.* 2012a, p.181). Staff were more likely to appreciate the IMHA's role if the advocate was considered to be effective in their role supporting service users or, indeed, if staff were already positively inclined towards advocacy in the first place. However, in some circumstances wherein staff were well disposed towards the advocates from the outset, the boundaries of independence were potentially jeopardised. Certain staff expressed how they felt that their clinical role was enhanced by the input of an IMHA who had more accurately elicited their patients' wants and needs. Thus, staff could ironically conceive of advocacy as something of an adjunct to the professionals, or an extension of team working: helpful for the team, if not quite a member of the team. In the extreme, these relations might appear to qualifying patients as too close or enmeshed, violating proper boundaries or co-opting advocacy.

Staff confusion regarding the place and importance of independent advocacy is not restricted to IMHA. In a study of staff understandings of advocacy in the learning disability context, there was limited appreciation of the differences between IMCA and other forms of advocacy and less than 50 per cent of care managers understood circumstances in which an IMCA referral would be appropriate (Martins *et al.* 2011).

Uneasy relations

Bateman (2000) has noted an ambiguity in disposition towards advocacy from health and welfare organisations, with perhaps diminishing enthusiasm when such advocacy is strong and effective. Brandon (1998), speaking from personal experience as both an advocate and survivor, described resistance from professionals coupled with a readiness to dismiss service users' demands as irrational or unreasonable as the main impediments to the assertion of advocacy as a serious potential contributor on the psychiatric scene. In the early years of UK advocacy practice, Sang and O'Brien (1984) were particularly sceptical of the possibility of providing advocacy within organisations where professionals were ill disposed to supporting advocacy. Conversely Ivers (1994, 1998) noted evidence that health care professionals warmed to the idea of citizen advocacy through recognising the positive contribution in the lives of those who by virtue of advocacy intercessions negotiated better support from services and hence became more satisfied with the service.

Mallik (1997) described the importance of affect, strong emotions or moral outrage in sustaining some nurses' identification with an advocacy role. This could be in a context of angrily objecting to care decisions seemingly grounded in economics rather than patients' wishes or needs, or as a challenge to perceived medical dominance. Both sets of circumstances raise the possibility of nurses' vulnerability when acting as advocates within established managerial or professional hierarchies.

Objection to medical dominance resonates with certain aspects of nursing's own professionalisation journey, and hence professional identity. To be denied a claim on such signifying roles therefore can be seen to be undermining of a positive sense of occupational identity, and may help to explain some of the complexity of nurses', and other professionals', discomfort with challenges posed by independent advocacy (McKeown *et al.* 2002).

Professionals' emotional response to advocacy might possibly be linked to wider experiences of alienation in their day-to-day work, including an alienated sense of selfhood that comes from systemic impediments to caring for others (Ferguson and Lavalette 2004; McKeown *et al.* 2010). For instance, in a study of nursing practice on acute in-patient wards in New Zealand, many of the nurses revealed their sense of powerlessness to effect change on behalf of patients: 'there is no professional fulfilment then…this gives the nurse no power so in a way it makes you feel quite worthless' (Fourie *et al.* 2005, p.138).

Nursing staff and others may prefer to project a positive image of their own role as carer rather than custodian, and a claim on an advocacy role is one means of realising this, or at least minimising some of the dissonant aspects of professional identity, beset with the obvious contradictions attendant on employment in a coercive system.

The negative disposition of some mental health staff towards advocacy may, however, be more prosaic and can be understood in simpler terms. For example, Ivers (1998) highlights the discomfort and intrusion that some professionals can experience with the presence of an advocate as a third person in the relationship with service users. Harrison and Davis (2009) hint at the possibility that some of the tensions between staff and advocates exist because advocacy interventions expose any disparities between what is actually available from services and what service users want to be provided. Whilst recognising this, professionals may feel powerless to make the changes or to secure the resources needed, and thus resentful of those outside the system 'interfering', as they see it. This perception can be extended to relations with family carers who undertake an advocacy role as well as independent advocates.

> Many professionals have achieved a great deal through promoting their patients' interests. It is important, though, to acknowledge that such advocacy carries with it the temptation to act on behalf of the people that they are working for and strong reliance on professional expertise and judgement. It is always best to encourage individuals to make their own case (self-advocate) and to assist them, for example, through independent advocacy in developing the skills to achieve this. (Harrison and Davis 2009, p.82)

The need for advocates to protect their independence and to create an appropriate distance or boundary between them and professional staff can leave staff feeling affronted or questioning of the relational skills of the advocate. In the extreme, working relations in these circumstances can become tense, hostile or even break down completely. Staff can become aggrieved or consider that the actions of the advocate call into question their professionalism, or they feel upset that service users appear to trust the advocate more than staff or have a better relationship with advocates (McKeown et al. 2002). Similarly, strenuous assertion of the value of independent advocacy also hints at the potential for causing discomfort in staff:

> Criticism is implicit in advocacy. If it is to highlight the many instances where people's needs are managed but not met, if it is to speak up for those who would otherwise be ignored, it cannot be part of the routine structures of care provision. Independence is for this reason the hallmark of true advocacy, for independence creates the space within which criticism can be formulated. (Henderson and Pochin 2001, p.153)

The sense that advocacy is unequivocally about criticism has been the basis of much disquiet amongst professional staff, who might equate criticism as inevitably potentiating complaints. Henderson and Pochin (2001), however, point out that criticism can also be about endorsement. Thus, in our study, whilst some staff were uncomfortable with being confronted, others viewed this as a good thing: 'We should be challenged, we need to be challenged, we should always be challenging the system for the benefit of the patient. We need to be kept on our toes' (AMHP/social worker quoted in Newbigging *et al.* 2012a, p.182). Other staff, however, would resist advocacy involvement and see advocates as interfering or there to cause trouble:

> There is this 'us and them', they're there to challenge us, they're there to cause problems, they're there to trip us up... you do get that sort of sense that you're under attack and so...you're on your guard...and if the nursing staff are feeling uncomfortable about people, they're not going to push it, you know they'll go through the form and tick the boxes. (Ward manager quoted in McKeown *et al.* 2014a, p.403)

A significant difference in outlook between many practitioner staff and advocates hinges upon staff pursuance of what they understand to be in the patient or service user's 'best interest'. The fact that advocates support people to express their view regardless of concern with best interest leads some staff to view them as unrealistic, naive or even irresponsible. On the contrary, staff who appreciate the advocacy role recognise that individuals will not always want what the clinical team think is in their best interests: for instance, higher doses of medication or being detained in hospital. Different perspectives between advocates and clinicians can surface in, for example, discussions of risk and the merits or otherwise of positive risk taking rather than risk-averse practices.

A matrix of working relations

Grounded in the findings of our study of IMHA and congruent with other research and commentary, we have developed a matrix that represents various aspects of the accounts of working relations between advocates and mental health staff (see Figure 11.1). The respective quadrants of this matrix correspond to different forms that the relationship might take between staff and advocates, influenced by the degree of understanding of the advocacy role or appreciation for advocacy on the part of the staff. Particular emotional reactions to advocacy are also associated with the interrelationship between knowledge and disposition depicted in each quadrant.

Previous experiences of advocacy (positive or negative) can shape current disposition. However, a prior negative experience of advocacy need not inevitably lead to a lasting antipathy. Advocates' efforts to develop better understandings and appreciation for advocacy can bear fruit and counter negative expectations over time. The fact that antagonistic relations existed in our study suggests that previously reported hostile or sceptical attitudes regarding advocacy's empowerment potential have proved obdurate (Gamble 1999; Tyrer 1989), and need positive and targeted actions such as regular awareness-raising sessions by advocates to dissipate.

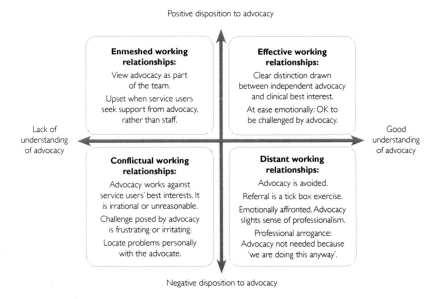

Figure 11.1 A matrix of working relationships

The top right-hand quadrant in the matrix accounts for the optimum, constructive working relations, where good understanding coincides with positive appreciation for the value of advocacy and the difference it can make to securing the best care and treatment for service users. To some degree, all of the forms represented in the other quadrants are less helpful and can be associated with poorer relations and outcomes. Enmeshed working relations result, for example, in circumstances where inadequate staff knowledge of the independence boundary in particular combines with a positive disposition, resulting in attempts to frame advocates as 'part of the team'. The distant and conflictual relationships share disregard for the value of advocacy, but differ in the degree of understanding of the nature of the independent advocacy role. Hence, it is relatively easy to engage in conflictual relations in circumstances where staff lack knowledge of advocacy in tandem with holding to the view that advocates are interfering or working against service users' best interests.

Positive relations

Mental health services play an important role in determining the quality and effectiveness of advocacy depending on the extent to which they offer appropriate support. Within these services, the right to access independent advocacy can be predicated upon mutual understanding and appreciation of role between practitioner and advocacy personnel. Carver and Morrison's (2005) small-scale study of the work of independent advocates in UK acute mental health wards developed insights into the nature of advocacy practice in these settings and stressed the importance of good-quality relationships between advocates and ward staff. Various studies, including our own, have made the case for effective boundaries in the working relations between staff and advocates that maintain the independence of advocacy. This can involve the advocates taking care to balance the need for positive, civil and constructive relationships with staff without appearing to get too close.

The fact that many staff fail to understand or appreciate the role of the advocates points to a need for better training of staff to be informed and prepared to support advocacy, although it should be acknowledged that such training does not guarantee eventual positive attitudes. In the same study, the advocates were very conscious of the need not to let the necessity of effective working relations with care teams compromise independence: 'Advocates were very aware that in developing good working relationships with staff they may compromise their independence or create the impression among clients they were part of the clinical team' (Carver and Morrison 2005, p.82).

Contemplating the potential for advocacy to perform a mediation function at times of crisis in the lives of advocacy partners, Craig and De Souza (1998, p.199) stress the positive contribution to 'interdisciplinary co-operative caregiving in supporting people in healthcare decision making'. In contrast, Brandon (1998, p.144) warned of the dangers of co-option: 'from being hated outsiders to becoming just another part of the service'. Fighting against resistance from services risks burnout for the advocates. Conversely, and perhaps presciently, Brandon (1998) anticipated other hazards in the future development of the advocacy role: 'As it gains power, influence and investment, there is a great danger of arid professionalization' (p.144), a theme to which we will return in our concluding chapter.

In our study, both positive and negative experiences of working relationships were reported from the perspectives of both advocates and mental health staff. The advocates put considerable effort into developing relationships and improving staff knowledge of the IMHA role. Indeed, in Chapter 9 we touched upon the need for IMHAs to develop good relationship skills, not just in order to relate effectively to a diverse range of qualifying patients, but to be able to operate effectively within complex mental health systems. This included taking care to establish trust and avoid the potential for staff to feel threatened by advocacy. The advocates' interpersonal skills, developed primarily for the advocacy relationship, were also invaluable and appreciated for building relationships with care teams (McKeown et al. 2013; Newbigging et al. 2014).

A rather obvious way forward would be the cooperative development of training initiatives, with mental health services and advocacy organisations, along with service users, working together to design and deliver appropriate training and associated resources. Such efforts would aim to improve understandings and appreciation of advocacy and model best practice in working relationships. Reference to the matrix could facilitate open and honest reflections on current working practices with a view to appreciating strengths and identifying room for improvement. With skilled facilitation, the various emotional reactions prompted by advocacy involvement could be aired and addressed. Our own implementation project in alliance with the Social Care Institute for Excellence has relied upon such stakeholder collaboration to co-produce a range of relevant resources, grounded in the findings of the research which are freely available (for further details see SCIE/UCLan 2015 in the Useful Resources section).

Martins and colleagues (2011) suggest that one solution for staff ignorance of advocacy that moves beyond the obvious strategy of training is to designate an advocacy champion within service teams, who becomes responsible for promoting better understanding of advocacy amongst colleagues. Without a doubt staff are capable of forming more appreciative understandings of advocacy, and we speculate whether such knowledge will deepen across services as new legally defined forms of advocacy persist and become more embedded over time. Similarly, Henderson *et al.* (2010) in a US study of advanced directives argued that there might be better results with more attention to the process of their completion and extending the implicit idea of consumer choice to receiving support from independent advocacy in this context.

Conclusions

Health and social care professionals' claim that advocacy is inherent to their professional role cannot be seen to replace the need for truly independent advocacy to support the service users' voice within disempowering systems. Despite such claims being bound up with a passionate concern with democratising the relations of health and social care service delivery, professionals need to recognise the limits of their ability to advocate from within systems, of their tendency towards best interests advocacy, and to recognise that they are often part of the problem and not just the solution. A limited view of advocacy and confusion over who can take on such a role in a mental health context contributes to strained working relationships between professionals and independent advocates. One person interviewed for the purposes of writing the history of Nottingham Advocacy Group points out that the relationship between advocacy organisations and service providers has always to some extent been an uneasy one, yet perhaps there is increasingly little doubt about the legitimate authority of advocacy:

> ...whereas a decade ago the idea that you might pay somebody to criticise you was like an alien concept. It is now almost like, again, come into the culture as any healthy organisation that has got nothing to hide except that it needs, that its users need some sort of advocacy, it has got to have a complaints procedure, and that you actually get brownie points now for buying advocacy as part of the package. (Anonymous interviewee, quoted in Barnes 2007, p.46)

The need for a healthy, mutually respectful and positive working culture to develop between mental health services and advocates is paramount for ensuring service users' rights are delivered within increasingly coercive settings. In practice these working relations will be shaped by the extent to which there can be shared understanding and sensible expectations of each other's roles. The matrix of working relationships developed from our research findings shows that where advocacy is understood *and* appreciated then effective working relationships will follow, and staff will face subsequent criticism or challenges with equanimity.

REFLECTIVE EXERCISES

1. Consider disposition to independent advocacy in the matrix of working relationships from the perspective of your own mental health service or from what you know of a local mental health service. Where does the service sit on the scale – is it positively or negatively predisposed to advocacy? What are the implications of this?

2. Again using the matrix of working relationships, think about local mental health staff's understanding of independent advocacy and its role. Is this good or poor, or somewhere in between? What are the implications of this for effective advocacy?

3. The matrix of working relationships summarises aspects of the relationships between advocacy services and mental health services that impact the effectiveness of advocacy. Could this be a useful tool to support professional and service development in practice, and if so, how would you use it?

4. Make a list of all the factors that influence the quality of relationships between IMHAs and mental health professionals. Then categorise or group these, for example individual professionals' attitudes, organisational culture, etc. What can you learn from this?

Chapter 12

COMMISSIONING EFFECTIVE INDEPENDENT MENTAL HEALTH ADVOCACY SERVICES

Introduction

This chapter looks critically at the commissioning of IMHA services and explores how improving the commissioning process can facilitate more accessible and appropriate IMHA services for all qualifying patients. Commissioning is entrenched in misunderstandings and often narrowly construed as a transactional process. In this chapter, we approach commissioning as a transformational process with the potential to shape outcomes for people using health and social care services and influence the wider system. However, commissioning is vulnerable to ideological shifts in welfare policy, not least the unprecedented cuts to local authority budgets seen since 2010.

In this chapter, we consider the role of commissioning in shaping IMHA services at a local level and in defining IMHA provision, and ensuring that service user-defined outcomes are met. We start by considering what commissioning is and what good commissioning looks like. Central to effective commissioning is co-production and co-design with people who have lived experience of compulsion, and we look at what co-production means in the context of commissioning IMHA services. The commissioning of IMHA services moved to local authorities in April 2013, and we reflect on the findings from a recent FOI request on the status of the current commissioning by local authorities since they took up this role. We conclude by considering the steps commissioners can take to promote the delivery of high-quality IMHA services, integrated with a range of other forms of advocacy and delivered in a mental health service context committed to promoting the rights of all service users.

The commissioning process

From our research, it was clear that participants considered commissioning played a critical role in the development of good-quality IMHA services and ensuring that everyone has access to an IMHA when they need one (Newbigging *et al.* 2012). The term 'commissioning' is still associated with compulsory competitive tendering, which was ushered in as part of the purchase–provider split in health and social care in the early 1990s (Bovaird, Dickinson and Allen 2012). As a consequence, it is often equated with procurement: a transactional process of identifying and contracting with a service provider to meet people's needs. Since 2004, commissioning in public services has increasingly been framed as a transformational process, 'in order to achieve outcomes for citizens, communities and society as a whole; based on knowing their needs, wants, aspirations and experience' (Bovaird *et al.* 2012; Cabinet Office 2013, p.4).

There are different models of commissioning and a wealth of guidance on standards, but relatively little evidence for the impact of effective commissioning (Health Services Management Centre (HSMC) 2014a). However, there is currently significant political investment in commissioning as a mechanism to improve the quality and impact of public services. The Care Act 2014 frames commissioning in terms of shaping the provision of care (i.e. the market), driving up quality and enabling citizens to manage their own lives and stay independent as long as possible. In a context of financial austerity the implicit motivation for this has been widely criticised for reducing public sector spending and reducing the role of the state. Nonetheless, it also represents a continued shift away from institutional models of care to enabling people to have greater choice and control over their care and support in response to service user demands.

Commissioning is often represented as a cyclical process of activity that involves engaging with individuals and communities; understanding assets and needs; defining outcomes and priorities; designing the solutions to address the identified needs, for example a service model; and action planning to achieve the agreed priorities and evaluating the impact of the action taken. In local government this is typically described as 'Analyse, Plan, Do, Review'. Post-positivist approaches to commissioning interpret this as a dynamic learning process and emphasise the role of values in shaping commissioning activity (Heginbotham 2012). Referred to as values-based commissioning, this places equal importance on service user and carer values and perspectives as professional expertise, and evidence from systematic studies.

Principles and standards developed to support high-quality commissioning generally (see HMSC 2014b), as summarised in Box 12.1, provide a framework for assessing the quality of IMHA service commissioning, alongside more bespoke guidance for commissioning advocacy (Newbigging *et al.* 2008; NIMHE 2008; SCIE 2014).

BOX 12.1 PRINCIPLES UNDERPINNING EFFECTIVE COMMISSIONING

The principles are:

- co-production with people using services, their carers and advocates

- clarity of purpose, focused on outcomes

- leadership and transparency

- equity

- personalisation

- joint commissioning between health and social care

- based on sound knowledge of need and evidence

- investment matched to need

- performance management focus on quality and outcomes

- developing providers to provide high-quality services

- developing commissioning competencies.

(Source: Adapted from Health Services Management Centre 2014b)

Commissioning in health and social care increasingly emphasises outcomes, and we looked at this in more detail in Chapter 8. However, this is no substitute to working with individuals, carers, service user groups and communities to define outcomes and evaluate that what matters most to them has been achieved (Farquharson 2014). Furthermore, current policy and legislation seek to shift the relationship between commissioners and providers from an adversarial relationship to one in which there is trust and transparency, articulated in the Care Act 2014, as a duty placed on local authorities of 'market shaping'. This language reflects the current ideology and embraces all providers of social care, including those commissioned by individuals through direct payments and personal budgets as well as large organisations providing services to many people, as with residential care.

Policy articulates a normative view of commissioning, with increasing emphasis on the market-shaping duty whose purpose is stated as ensuring there are high-quality services available to meet local needs and to drive up the quality of this provision. The implicit task, however, is to balance current policy and law with the aspirations of local people, communities and politicians, the available evidence and good practice within finite resources to achieve the best-quality services for this investment. Inevitably this involves prioritising the use of available resources, and increasingly commissioners are required to be transparent about this process and the decisions they are making.

Co-production and commissioning

The term co-production dates from the 1970s and more recently became a new way of describing working in partnership with people using services, carers, families and citizens. The interest in co-production across the full range of public services, not just social care and health, is motivated partly by financial pressures on local authorities but is also indicative of the widespread acknowledgement that the citizen has a vital role in achieving positive public service outcomes (Ostrom 1996). Co-production builds on participation and involvement models. In co-production, people who use services are involved right from the start as equal partners, underpinned by a reciprocal relationship between service users, carers and professionals. It is defined by the SCIE Co-production Critical Friends group as 'a relationship where professionals and citizens share power to plan and deliver support together, recognising that both have vital contributions to make in order to improve quality of life for people and communities' (SCIE 2013). Co-production can be seen as a set of values, as summarised in Box 12.2, and an essential strand of a values-based approach to commissioning.

BOX 12.2 PRINCIPLES UNDERPINNING CO-PRODUCTION

Equality – everyone has assets: Co-production starts from the idea that no one group or person is more important than anyone else and everyone has skills, abilities and time to contribute.

Diversity: Co-production should be as inclusive and diverse as possible. Particular efforts may be needed to ensure that seldom-heard groups are included.

Accessibility: Making everything accessible is the way to ensure that everyone has an equal opportunity to participate fully in an activity in the way that suits them best.

Reciprocity: Reciprocity means people get something back for putting something in. There are formal ways of doing this, like using time banks as a way of rewarding people, but sometimes the reciprocity comes from the more equal relationships that develop between people and organisations.

(Source: Adapted from SCIE 2013)

Co-production can help ensure that resources are used to develop the services that people really want and are, therefore, linked with better outcomes for service users and carers. Co-designing IMHA services with service users, specifically people who have experience of compulsion, will both enable commissioners to identify the key outcomes to achieve for people and design a service that is able to provide a personalised response. This is of critical importance in developing IMHA services that service users have trust in and are, therefore, more likely to access, and reflects the foundational principles of advocacy.

Co-producing IMHA services with people that reflect the whole population, including seldom-heard groups, also means that barriers to access and issues relating to the style and organisation of local advocacy services can be addressed so that provision is culturally appropriate (Hakim and Pollard 2011; Newbigging *et al.* 2012a; Rai-Atkins *et al.* 2002). This means going beyond inclusion of the 'usual suspects' and also requires sufficient attention be paid to the diversity of the local population, age appropriateness and the likely need for non-instructed advocacy.

For co-production to be effective in commissioning, attention will need to be paid to:

- organisational culture and values: building an organisational culture on a shared understanding of what co-production means, how it is done and what will be achieved

- involving people who use services and carers from the start, valuing and rewarding everyone who takes part and ensuring there are resources to cover the cost of co-production

- ensuring everyone has the information, support and resources needed to be part of co-production and decision making and providing training for everyone in co-production and any other skills they will need

- regularly reviewing to ensure that co-production is making a real difference and that the process is following the agreed principles and using the findings to refresh and support continuous learning.

(Fleischman 2014)

The following provides a practical checklist for commissioners:

- Put systems in place to enable people who use services and carers to participate in commissioning in a meaningful way.

- Involve people who use services and carers in the design, development and monitoring of services.

- Involve people who use services (including current and former IMHA partners) and carers in the commissioning and tendering process.

- Involve service users and carers in contract monitoring.

- Provide appropriate ongoing support to enable co-production in commissioning.

- Ensure there are methods in place to enable IMHA partners to provide feedback on their experience to commissioners.

(SCIE/UCLan 2015b)

Co-producing advocacy services also increases the opportunities for advocacy organisations to interface with service user-led initiatives, for example peer support and support groups. It potentially opens up a conversation about the contribution of collective advocacy and goes some way to supporting a collectivist approach to promoting rights and lobbying for improvements in mental health care and treatment.

Commissioning IMHA services

The MH Act 2007 required that PCTs, who were responsible for commissioning health services for the local population, should make IMHA services available for qualifying patients. As noted earlier, Hakim and Pollard (2011) found wide variations in practice, with evidence of some good commissioning and provision in some areas and some PCTs that had not funded sufficient advocacy to meet the local needs or diverted funding from other advocacy services to commission IMHA services. They found particular gaps in relation to provision for people from BAME communities, reflected in the pace of introduction of IMHA services and the practice of continuing to contract with existing providers, both of which disadvantaged BAME organisations. By 2011, many PCTs were retendering for the provision of IMHA services but surprisingly, in our study there was little evidence of a dedicated needs assessment for IMHA services and, therefore, a lack of consideration of the specific advocacy needs of particular groups. A dedicated needs assessment is important as a basis for determining the service to be commissioned and the level of investment required. The issue of whether or not IMHA services are being adequately funded has been consistently raised and whether funding for other forms of advocacy (i.e. non-statutory) were being cut, with Action for Advocacy (2011) estimating that up to 66,000 people could be affected by these cuts.

Commissioning IMHA services became the responsibility of local authorities in 2013, through the Health and Social Care Act 2012. In a context of financial austerity, there is considerable pressure on public services, particularly local authorities, to reduce their costs, and other forms of non-statutory advocacy are likely to be at risk unless a clear case can be made for their continued survival. In summer 2014, we made a FOI request to all local authorities in England to ask about their commissioning of IMHA services to ascertain the status of commissioning post the Health and Social Care Act 2012. The response rate to the FOI request within the timeframe for the study was 69 per cent, and revealed different arrangements for commissioning IMHA services operating across England. Just under half reported that the commissioning of IMHA services is being undertaken by a single local authority (n = 51). Twenty-three local authorities reported that they were jointly commissioning with local CCGs and 15 reported that that the local authorities was commissioning on behalf of other local authorities or on behalf of one or more CCGs. In 11 local authorities the CCG commissions the IMHA service, reflecting historical arrangements or local agreement. The level of service user involvement, despite the promotion of co-production as good practice, was disappointing in our original study, and scant evidence this identified in the FOI research.

Defining the purpose of IMHA services

Local authority commissioners are working in difficult times when the pressures on local authority budgets and increased concerns about the quality of care and risks to vulnerable people will undoubtedly influence local decisions. As discussed within Chapter 3, the foundational principles of advocacy emphasise the importance of empowerment, and increasingly this is being framed within a rights discourse. The inclusion of advocacy in statutes means that at the very least this will have to be provided in order to avoid legal challenges. This places commissioners in a challenging position, where they may want to invest in advocacy in order to promote empowerment but only have the resources to ensure that statutory provisions are met. As two commissioners involved in our implementation project observed:

> A key decision will be whether the IMHA service is focused solely on the minimum legal requirement or the extent to which it will take a holistic perspective by setting wider empowering outcomes. This will be determined by the commissioning strategy and, in these constrained financial times, by budgetary realities. (Pringle and Lewis 2014)

This tension, and the factors which may influence its resolution, is illustrated in Figure 12.1. This may well challenge the spirit of co-production, with service users and carers arguing for a commissioning framework that allows the IMHA service to support people to achieve their outcomes, which as discussed in Chapter 5 are often broader than a narrow construction of upholding rights under the MH Act. Difficulties in balancing aspirations with the financial and political context may well be played out through explicit prioritisation in commissioning objectives and implicit gatekeeping by designing services that limit access, by IMHA providers prioritising particular people or by professionals limiting who they refer to the service: a form of street-level bureaucracy in a context of finite resources (Lipsky 1980).

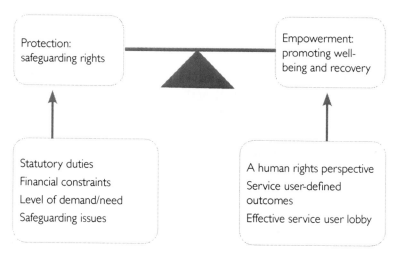

Figure 12.1 Factors influencing the definition of purpose of IMHA services by commissioners

Assessing needs for IMHA services

Needs assessment provides a foundation for ensuring that the IMHA services that are commissioned are appropriate for the whole community (Hakim and Pollard 2011). The needs assessment should cover:

- a profile of the local population and inequalities relevant to mental health

- an understanding of advocacy needs for people subject to compulsion

- an assessment of gaps in provision and opportunities to embed advocacy within a broader rights-based approach

- the experience and intelligence from current advocacy providers

- experience and intelligence from mental health service providers

- research and practice-based evidence on effective models for the delivery of advocacy services for people subject to compulsion.

Overall, commissioners have some way to go in ensuring advocacy provision is based on relevant and robust needs assessments. The mismatch between the provision of mental health advocacy and needs at a local level, first identified by Foley and Platzer (2007), has been confirmed by subsequent studies and in relation to IMHA (CQC 2015a), with those requiring advocacy being most likely to miss out (Hakim and Pollard 2011; Newbigging *et al.* 2012a). Despite attention having previously been drawn to the paucity of needs assessments, less than one in five of the local authorities responding to the FOI request in 2014 reported that they had undertaken one. Of those that had, some were overly general and did not identify the specific issues that particular groups might encounter, for example disproportionate detention of people from BAME communities, as discussed in Chapter 10.

A good-quality needs assessment will pick up the specific issues for the provision of IMHA services. This will include issues relating to demand, characteristics of the population being detained, and the recognition that some people might be detained more than once during a year. Our study also highlighted a difference in the rate of detentions between urban and rural areas, with the former having much higher rates of detention and significantly larger populations from BAME communities. The turnover in such circumstances may be more rapid, and this will have implications for the organisation of IMHA provision. Access in secure settings appears to be more straightforward because the population of qualifying patients is more static. Access to IMHA for people on CTOs, with increasing numbers particularly from BAME groups, has been identified as problematic (Stroud *et al.* 2013), and the needs assessment should include this group of people, as well as the relatively small numbers of people on guardianship orders. Demographic changes including a growing number of older people with dementia raises issues about the increased need for provision of non-instructed IMHA. Further more, specific consideration needs to be given to people with learning disabilities, deaf people and children and young people, all of whom are likely to require a different style of service.

Needs assessments are typically undertaken in relation to the local population, but it is evident that there has been considerable confusion and concern regarding IMHA provision for people placed out of their ordinary area of residence, usually in a secure unit frequently provided by the independent sector (CQC 2015a). In our study there was an instance where both a local commissioner and a commissioner from the person's place of residence – 200 miles away – were commissioning different advocacy services to provide an IMHA service to the individual. A wider survey of independent sector providers found a substantial number were commissioning their own IMHA services: a pragmatic response to the lack of clarity but compromising the principle of independence (Newbigging *et al.* 2012a). The revised Code of Practice makes it clear that local commissioners should commission for all qualifying patients detained in units in their locality (Department of Health 2015).

Developing a service model

The fulcrum of commissioning is developing a service model, and in an ideal world this should determine the level of investment as opposed to identifying the resources available and then shoehorning local stakeholders' aspirations and expectations for a service into the available financial resources. Commissioners have difficult decisions to make about resource allocation and prioritisation, but at the very least these need to be transparent and what is not possible should be made clear. The design of the service model should address the outcomes defined by service users with experience of compulsion and build on the intelligence collected from the needs assessment. A central question for commissioners, identified in our study, is whether IMHA services should be designed on the presumption that all people subject to compulsion should have access to an IMHA. This clearly reflects the spirit of the law and has become known as 'opt-out'. In other words, qualifying patients would be automatically referred to the IMHA service on detention and have to positively decide to decline the offer of an IMHA, the current arrangement being that qualifying patients have to refer themselves or be referred to the service. The opt-out arrangement (see SCIE/UCLan 2015 in the Useful Resources section) was recommended as a practical solution to the various barriers to access described previously and including implicit gatekeeping by professionals discussed in Chapter 11. This has profound implications for the design and investment in services, and requires consideration of data protection issues. A case study illustrating one approach to redesigning the local service to introduce a single point of access and an opt-out model is illustrated in Box 12.3.

BOX 12.3 COMMISSIONING IMHA SERVICES: A CASE STUDY

Lancashire County Council assumed responsibility for commissioning IMHA and redesigning advocacy provision (serving a total population of 1.3 million people), building on findings of the 'Right to be Heard' research.

Co-production

User representatives were initially engaged in June 2012 through a UCLan conference presenting recommendations of the IMHA research, and were subsequently involved in the commissioning process from October 2012. Invitations were sent to partnership boards, service user forums, carers and BAME organisations, and participants shaped the future of advocacy services by voicing their opinions on a series of questions. Feedback was used to influence service specifications and set further questions and scenarios in the tender questionnaire. Service user representatives, including from seldom-heard groups, were fully engaged in shortlisting and scoring applications from advocacy providers, and recommending contract awards.

Service model

The advocacy landscape has been simplified for both staff and the public by creating a **Single Point of Access** and encouraging all advocacy providers to work together to ensure all those eligible are able to access appropriate services. Lancashire County Council (LCC), as the lead commissioner, Lancashire Care Foundation Trust (LCFT) and Advocacy Focus, the new provider, have worked in partnership to develop a vision for IMHA services and overcome obstacles. An **Opt-out** system has been introduced for IMHA, operationalised as an **Open Advocacy Protocol** by LCFT, with a suite of podcasts launched at www.lancashire care.nhs.uk/about-us/Mental-Health-Act-Information.php.

The protocol clarifies roles and responsibilities for an opt-out advocacy model, from provision of information, making a referral, sharing information, and optimising learning from good practice through quarterly monitoring.

Impact of the new service model

- Equity of service regardless of deprivation/geographical restrictions and ethnicity. During the first year Advocacy Focus handled 1130 enquiries; 42 per cent of these were from people requesting support and 35 per cent were referrals for generic advocacy and IMHA.

- Access to IMHA has improved: the number of IMHA referrals has more than doubled from 404 in 2012/13 to 848 in 2013/14.

- Elimination of some practical problems faced by clinicians in making service users aware of their rights (when they are extremely unwell or unable to comprehend) or whether or not to refer when faced with people lacking capacity.

- Additional safeguards for service users who are unable to communicate or assert themselves to uphold their basic rights and entitlements through a new non-instructed contract.

- Improved relationships, communication and engagement with Mental Health Act administrators/ LCFT staff and advocacy providers, enabling individuals to have increased choice and control in having their voice heard. Regular advocacy presence on the wards provides opportunities for service users to indicate a need for advocacy at any time during their stay.

- Continuity of advocacy support for individuals transferring from generic advocacy to IMHA on wards and vice versa, as advocates are designated to a hospital and have regular presence.

- Due to its success, LCFT is considering extending this model to older adults and secure mental health services.

Challenges faced

- Lack of understanding of the role of IMHA and non-instructed advocacy amongst staff, requiring further training.

- Varying interpretations of the information to be shared across hospitals in Lancashire and the potential for duplicate referrals from several sources initially led to increased advocacy staff time to eliminate these. This has been overcome through sharing concerns and staff double checking records prior to referral.

- The consistency and regularity of information to notify the provider service of patients requiring an IMHA, improved through regular meetings and reports.

- Sharing of information without breaching confidentiality/data protection by omitting names of individuals who objected to having an IMHA; all others that were able/unable to instruct were referred with initials.

- Future development and planning via twice-yearly Strategic Advocacy Meetings which involve NHS and local government commissioners, providers and user representatives, and information is also shared with Local Healthwatch.

(Source: Angela Esslinger, Lancashire County Council)

Service specifications that reflect local needs assessments are often taken as the hallmark of commissioning quality IMHA services (National Mental Health Development Unit 2009a; Newbigging *et al.* 2012a), as they describe in detail the expectations of the service in terms of how it will operate and the outcomes that it will achieve. However, as of 2014, just under two-thirds of local authorities indicated that they had a service specification, leaving open the question about the basis on which they will be able to monitor the IMHA service. A quarter of the local authorities were commissioning IMHA services only, although it is likely that the advocacy service was providing a broader range of advocacy and it was evident in some instances that the single contract was additional to a contract for generic mental health advocacy with another local authority or CCG. However, commissioning statutory advocacy only (i.e. IMHA/IMCA, DOLS and NHS complaints advocacy, or combinations of these) was reported by 59 per cent of the commissioners who provided information in this regard. A significant number of local authorities are commissioning the full range of statutory advocacy alongside non-statutory advocacy, typically referred to as generic advocacy but usually for people experiencing mental health issues (n = 39).

Investment in IMHA services

The issue of whether or not IMHA services are being adequately funded was raised in our study, and the absence of robust needs assessment leaves the definitive answer to this question open. Investment, in addition to the costs of face-to-face contact, is necessary to support organisational capacity and outreach work and to build partnerships with community groups and relationships with mental health services to support the provision of effective IMHA services, including:

- costs of interpreters

- IMHA training and upskilling community organisations to deliver IMHA services

- training and raising awareness of mental health staff

- administrative and management costs associated with data collection for service monitoring

- publicity and promotion, particularly outreach to in-patient wards

- travel and travelling time, an issue for services covering large rural areas.

In recognition of this, the practice of spot purchasing and 'earned income' was seen by IMHA services as problematic and as compromising continuity and stability of provision as well as the capacity of IMHA services to provide outreach and promote access.

As discussed earlier, the investment in all statutory forms of advocacy, including the new requirement of the Care Act 2014, is likely to impact on investment in other forms of advocacy or to constrain the operation of IMHA to the statutory function only. This would not be consistent with service user views or the recommendations of the advocacy sector. Furthermore, the only study to compare different forms of advocacy (Rosenman et al. 2000) identified that the style of advocacy – personalised versus legal advocacy – had an impact on outcomes, including reduced lengths of stay in hospital and rehospitalisation (see Chapter 6 for more detail). In a context of joint commissioning between local authorities and CCGs, the benefits of investment in a whole system of advocacy will be more readily understood than when the local authority is the sole commissioner and, thus, the consequences of commissioning decisions and their impact on health spending less evident. Advocacy services have, therefore, argued for standardisation to guide local commissioning decisions, including resourcing as well as service specifications, in respect of IMHA to address potential inequities and mismatch between need and provision. In our study, the value of the national formula for IMCA services, which although described as imperfect, was appreciated for its transparency and its contribution to facilitating local service developments.

Tendering and contracting

There is increasing concern that tendering practice privileges large providers and, therefore, that locally valued providers are being squeezed out (see for example Brown, Standen and Khilji 2013). Thus, there are fears that the current climate of competition, rather than raising the quality of provision, may lead to costs being curtailed:

> I guess development will be hindered because there's this constant bid and competition for funding, which means services are trying to undercut other services when they apply for a contract, which means at the end services are actually going to start going downhill because people will be saying 'well I can do 18 wards with just one part time Advocate' because they're desperate to have the contract so the quality is going to go down with all this competition unless there's like a standardised I guess sort of requirement from Commissioners as to what kind of service needs to be provided. (IMHA quoted in Newbigging *et al.* 2012a, p.214)

Larger organisations are often better placed to respond to tenders as they have a more developed infrastructure for responding and can achieve economies of scale, meaning that on the face of it they appear to represent better value for money. However, this does not necessarily mean that they will provide a locally responsive service. As discussed in Chapter 7, the FOI request indicated that the type of organisations being commissioned varied, with national organisations covering large parts of England in the majority. Broadly speaking, these were of two types: either national organisations focused on mental health providing a range of services including accommodation, or they were specifically providing a range of advocacy. Commissioners were also commonly commissioning organisations that covered a geographical area, for example a county or parts of England – the south west, for instance. Commissioning local organisations, some of which were affiliated to a national organisation, such as Mind, was also occurring but less frequently, raising questions about the future direction of commissioning for IMHA services.

BAME and other advocacy providers for marginalised communities are, therefore, at risk in tendering processes not only because of their size but also if commissioners lack a developed understanding of the needs of diverse BAME communities, arising from inadequate needs assessment and different conceptions of advocacy. Furthermore we have found little evidence that commissioners are undertaking equality analysis, as part of the tendering process, as required by the Equality Act 2010. Commissioners can also be constrained by risk-averse rules for procurement, inherently leading commissioners down a path towards more established services. Accessible and proportionate processes for commissioning, funding and regulation will enable small community-based providers to contribute to the spectrum of provision (Carr 2014).

In both our study and our later FOI request, findings indicate that typically the length of the contracts awarded tend to be from one to three years. The level of investment reported by local authorities ranged from £26,000 to over half a million, but it is not possible to make meaningful comparisons in terms of investment in IMHA services on the basis of the available data, as it was often unclear what the expenditure related to in terms of service or time period. If local authority commissioners continue to be required to make financial savings, they will seek to reduce the transactional costs of commissioning, and this is likely to incentivise them to contract with larger organisations.

When commissioning organisations go out to tender and there is a change of provider, IMHAs will often move to the new provider, under Transfer of Undertakings Protection of Employment (TUPE) regulations, and these processes of transition need to be well managed, not only for staff but also for service users. There is a tendency for the focus to shift to the complexities of service reorganisation and away from service delivery without careful thought and preparation.

Monitoring arrangements

On the basis of our study and the FOI request, it appears the majority of commissioners have monitoring arrangements in place and require activity data to be provided, usually on a quarterly basis. This tends to relate to the activity of the service, but in some instances IMHA services have provided individual case studies or undertaken SROI assessment, although this tends to be for the range of advocacy provision rather than IMHA specifically. However, there needs to be methods for evaluating access to enable commissioners, and wider groups, to understand whether people's right to an IMHA is being upheld.

Obtaining data on outcomes is more difficult, for the reasons we discuss in Chapter 8, and requires information from mental health providers, which may not be readily available, particularly when commissioning is not undertaken jointly by health and local authorities. Information from IMHA services is valuable not only for the commissioning of IMHA services but also for commissioning mental health, and wider health and social care, services.

Implications for commissioning mental health services

Ensuring a positive relationship between the advocacy provider and the mental health secondary care provider is critical to the effective operation of IMHA services, as discussed in the previous chapter. There is a clear need for ongoing training and awareness raising of the service so that staff are clear when to refer to it. This is especially important when opt-out arrangements are not in place, to ensure that all those who qualify for the service are made aware of it, and where service users lack capacity and so require a referral to be made on their behalf. Specific training requirements relate to staff's understanding of the interface between the MH Act and the MC Act but also of the general role of advocates in representing the person's views and the difference from a 'best interests' approach.

The importance of mental health services being monitored on activity in relation to IMHA services and their responsibility in facilitating access to IMHA support has been recognised by the Care Quality Commission (CQC 2015a). In commissioning the service it needs to be recognised that there is a potential for tension between advocates and the secondary care provider. By building standard requirements into the contracts with mental health service providers, a positive organisational context can be established for the IMHA service to operate within. Training of mental health staff will help to ensure a fuller understanding of the role of the advocate and help reduce any potential for misunderstanding or conflict.

Conclusions

As local authorities now have responsibility for commissioning all forms of statutory advocacy, as discussed in Chapter 4 there is an opportunity to develop a whole-system approach to advocacy, with different forms of statutory advocacy sitting alongside other forms of advocacy – peer advocacy, community advocacy, citizen advocacy and self-advocacy. It follows from the previous discussion that if commissioners are committed to commissioning as a transformational process that has the potential to change the experience of people detained under the MH Act, they need to take a number of steps to commission IMHA as part of a whole system of advocacy, as summarised in Box 12.4.

BOX 12.4 TOP TIPS FOR COMMISSIONERS

1.   Develop an awareness of the experiences of people subject to compulsion within which to locate your understanding of the role and responsibilities of IMHA and other forms of advocacy.

2.   Take a co-production approach to commissioning, which fully involves service users and carers.

3.   Develop IMHA services that meet the needs of communities by conducting an annual needs assessment and an equality impact assessment specific to advocacy and IMHA.

4.   Develop IMHA services that deliver meaningful outcomes for IMHA partners, reflecting what matters most to people subject to compulsion under the Act.

5.   Work with individuals and groups from diverse, and seldom-heard, communities to ensure that IMHA services are culturally sensitive and ensure equity of access.

6. Work with IMHA services to ensure that IMHA provision meets the needs of IMHA partners, and invest to develop capacity.

7. Invest in and support a whole systems approach to advocacy, linking IMHA to other forms of advocacy to ensure continuity of support to IMHA partners.

8. Ensure that IMHA services offer both instructed and non-instructed IMHA, and that the interface with IMCA and DOLS is clear.

9. Ensure that the IMHA service is adequately funded to support people placed locally from out of the area.

10. Work with CCG commissioners to ensure that the mental health service context in which IMHA services are delivered understand the role, facilitate access to IMHA services, and make adjustments to enable the effective delivery of IMHA services.

(Source: Adapted from SCIE/UCLan, 2015
– see the Useful Resources section)

The foundation for any action is co-production with people with experience of being subject to compulsion and ideally of IMHA services. The first step is likely to involve building an awareness of the right to access IMHA services, and commissioners will, therefore, need to consider the overall investment in promoting service user agency and the adoption of a rights-based and recovery-focused approach by local services.

Defining service user outcomes as described in Chapter 8 will provide a framework for identifying what matters to people, and to ensure that this is reflected in the commissioning process. In a context of financial austerity, generic forms of advocacy including community-based advocacy and peer advocacy are likely to be increasingly squeezed, with the tendency for commissioners to commission statutory advocacy only, validating the concerns of advocates in our study. The risks of this to facilitating inclusion and recovery need to be understood and debated.

REFLECTIVE EXERCISES

1. Identify the different steps that commissioners should take to ensure that all people qualifying for an IMHA know their right to access one, and that they have access to an IMHA should they want one. Is this happening in your local area?

2. Research your local commissioning process to answer the following questions: How is IMHA commissioned? Is open access operating? How effective is this in ensuring equitable access to IMHA services?

3. Design a commissioning process that involves co-production with qualifying patients and local service user organisations. Who needs to be involved locally? What needs to happen to ensure meaningful involvement in commissioning IMHA services?

4. Devise a measure of effectiveness in the commissioning of IMHA services. What would this look like?

Chapter 13

THE FUTURE FOR INDEPENDENT ADVOCACY

A Glass Half Full?

Introduction

The establishment of IMHA has brought into sharp focus concerns regarding the professionalisation and legitimacy of advocacy. The recent expansion of mental health advocacy in an independent, paid model is, however, perceived by many to have raised the profile of (mental health) advocacy for the good and has certainly fuelled interest in the role and impact of advocacy. These trends need to be understood in the context of mental health advocacy's roots in the service user movement, with implications for who should and should not legitimately be an advocate. Furthermore, the question of legitimacy, though it can plausibly be posed of advocacy, is primarily an ongoing concern for the psychiatric system that calls into being the need for independent advocates in the first place.

In this final chapter we aim to contribute further to these debates, reaffirming our affinity for effective access to, and provision of, high-quality advocacy (based on the evidence provided in this book), but also posing critical questions regarding the real effect of advocacy upon people's experience of coercive services. In this sense, we return to our golden thread, envisioning circumstances in which service users' voices are more completely heard and their human rights properly promoted and preserved. Advocacy can have its legitimacy questioned on two broad fronts. First, the psychiatric system and staff working within it can doubt the value or need for advocacy. From this standpoint, different forms of advocacy may be viewed as more or less illegitimate. That said, staff resistance to advocacy is not endemic and many mental health practitioners are genuine and enthusiastic supporters who readily see the value of an independent challenge. Second, and perhaps more fundamentally, the impact and wider social function of advocacy can be called into question. From this perspective, advocacy's contribution to emancipation is viewed as lacking credibility. Ultimately, the legitimacy of advocacy in a mental health context will be proven when the transformational aspirations of founding activists are realised. Until such time, advocates (professional or otherwise) are cautioned to take reflective stock of their individual and collective achievements. Any rational, honest judgment must properly appraise impact on both the lives of individual advocacy partners and, more generally, on the nature and conduct of the psychiatric system itself. Furthermore, as Macadam *et al.* (2013) concluded, the lack of robust evidence about advocacy's effectiveness, particularly its cost effectiveness, leaves it in a potentially vulnerable position in these difficult financial times.

The value of advocacy: ensuring voice and rights?

As we argued in Chapter 3, advocacy cannot be divorced from service user activism and wider civil rights movements. Clearly development of advocacy has not occurred within a vacuum, and a backdrop of ideological framings, mental health service configurations, policy promptings and legislative turns have all had a profound influence (see Chapter 4). Any conception of IMHA has to be understood within the legal system grounded in a liberal western polity which has consistently emphasised rights, although their inclusiveness of people with mental health problems has been contested. More recently still, a populist countervailing bandwagon for an abrogation from rights charters has been leapt upon by some governments – including our own – dressed up as a defence of individualism and personal freedom from state interference. Such agile ideological gymnastics are less of a paradox if we consider the influence of neoliberalism and the undoubted fact that mental health services, and associated legislation, have been designed less to serve the interests of patients and more to protect the public from perceived risk (Rogers and Pilgrim 2014).

A robust defence of service users' rights insists upon the importance of independence from statutory provision, this being one of the foundational principles of all forms of advocacy. For people subject to compulsion, if their rights are to be protected, then everyone needs to have the opportunity to access an advocate. As has been discussed in previous chapters, the commissioning arrangements, mental health service staff's attitudes, lack of understanding of the role of IMHA by people subject to detention and ways of working that fail to reach out to specific sections of the population can all variously conspire to compromise this aspiration.

Mental health services have an important role to play in shaping the context for the delivery of IMHA services. The best outcomes will occur where staff both understand and value the advocacy role, particularly independence (see Chapter 11). The translation of aspirations for advocacy into practice is optimised when commissioners understand, value and invest in services that are accessible (see Chapter 12). As we have seen in Chapter 10, an effective 'inverse care law' may operate, whereby those who need advocacy the most get it least. Hence it behoves commissioners and allies of advocacy to plan and appropriately fund services based on a systematic appraisal of need and appreciation of the challenges facing some service users in making themselves heard.

Demonstrating the value of advocacy is an important consideration when legitimacy is at stake, but to date there have been relatively few robust studies, and even less that have involved service users in the research process. Again, this is neglectful of a heritage in survivor activism. What is more, advocates themselves are not necessarily involved in the conception, planning or conduct of research into advocacy, and are perhaps even less likely to be involved than service users. This perhaps reflects a move away from its roots in the survivor and user movement.

It may also reflect the current trajectory of advocacy, being a fairly immature profession in comparison with those that are more archetypal or established. A mark of a more mature profession would, for example, be the establishment of an academic field to mirror the practice discipline, including higher-level education opportunities and a self-defined research agenda.

For many service users, the value of advocacy is appreciated and for some it has been life changing, as Kris makes clear in his foreword. However, key research findings suggest that people can be more satisfied with the process rather than the outcomes of advocacy. That is, advocacy intervention is very much appreciated, and may be a pleasant contrast with routine experiences of care, but the tangible wishes of service users are not necessarily realised. This raises an important critique of initiatives like advocacy or models of service user involvement that aspire to emancipatory ends (Cooke and Kothari 2002). In a context of wider concern regarding the role of health care services within systems of governance and social control, is advocacy able to transform services or does it merely serve to pacify disgruntled or aggrieved individuals, restoring order in the system and effectively preserving the status quo? (McKeown et al. 2013.)

In a context of shrinking resources, commissioners and others also need to be alert to the perils of street-level bureaucracy (Lipsky 1980), with front-line workers potentially controlling matters of resource distribution and access regardless of the intentions of planners and policy makers. Such concerns illustrate some of the potential benefits and pitfalls of a professional advocacy identity, the quest for which is at least one dimension of enhancing legitimacy (Harrison and Davis 2009).

Professionalisation: perils and possibilities?

Arguments for and against advocates seeking greater professional status have been rehearsed both within the ranks of mental health advocates and service users. The very idea of professionalisation opens up consideration of both possibilities and perils for advocacy. The values, knowledge and skills of IMHAs are paramount to effective and valued practice. The key characteristics are well rehearsed and include rights-based, non-judgmental foundations for the exercise of high-quality relational skills with an understanding of the territory in which they are operating and in particular the impact of compulsions on people's lives (see Chapter 9). Arguably, an uncritical adoption of a mission to professionalise is in tension with some of the fundamental advocacy values, not least the potential to create 'professional' distance between advocates and their advocacy partners.

Debates about professionalism are not unique to advocacy, and have figured in the histories of many emerging occupational groups that have aspired to professional status. These include other groups of mental health workers, such as nurses. Sociologists of work have studied the professionalisation of various groups and the extent to which others are seemingly excluded from 'full' professional status (see Etzioni 1969). The acceptance or rejection of aspiring members of the professional 'club' has been analysed with reference to a number of factors, all of which are arguably relevant to advocacy's positioning as an occupational group:

- the economics of employment

- the transaction of power between various occupational groups

- the transaction of power between professionals and service users

- the importance of forms of social stratification such as class and gender.

The notion of advocacy seeking professional status has arguably happened by stealth and not necessarily always under the control of advocates. Nevertheless, our study suggests there is less resistance to this identification with professionalism amongst IMHAs compared with earlier disquiet expressed by advocates operating in different circumstances within different forms of advocacy. In this regard, advocates may look simultaneously in two directions: at one and the same time, happy to pursue the possibility of greater esteem from other professionals and associated remuneration, but also concerned not to in some way spoil the balance of their relationships with service users or to depart from core values (see Table 13.1).

TABLE 13.1 POSITIVE AND NEGATIVE ASPECTS OF THE PROFESSIONALISATION OF ADVOCACY	
Positive aspects	**Negative aspects**
• Credibility with other disciplines. • Improved self-image. • Enhanced status and esteem. • Improved pay. • Associated with training opportunities. • Perception of doing a 'professional' job of work; doing a good job. • Accountability. • Accreditation and regulation of practice. • Limiting entry to the profession – keeping out incompetent individuals. • Ownership of the title 'advocacy'.	• Connotations of elitism. • Establishes distance from service users. • Negative image of archetypal professions. • Tendency to disempowering practices, such as use of technical language/jargon. • Accommodation or incorporation into the mental health system. • Lose sight of place of service user's agenda as central focus. • Association with issue of central, public funding – threatens independence.

The quest for professional status often involves a desire to be associated with the positive trappings of established professions such as esteem, credibility and a sense of legitimacy.

However, occupational groups who also wish to be perceived as caring and supportive allies of service users are often simultaneously wary of taking on board some of the more unwholesome aspects of the established professions. Interwoven with these concerns are further worries that a too simplistic dash for professional status risks some key and valued features of the advocacy role, such as independence from services and care team personnel.

This duality in disposition towards the trappings of certain archetypal professions such as law and medicine has been mirrored in the professionalisation strategies of other occupational groups, such as nursing and social work. These aspects of the sociology of work offer the new profession of advocacy some potential food for thought. For instance, critical commentators like Davies (1996) invoke feminist analyses of the practices of 'masculinist' professionals. It is argued that it is not necessarily professionalisation in itself which is flawed, but which particular version of professionalism is aspired to. Davies (1996) argues for a reconstructed professionalism for nurses. The extrapolation of this is an actual transformation of the power within services with opportunities for alternative forms of care and treatment and robust challenges to epistemic injustices.

Legitimacy and epistemic justice

If professionalisation is one means by which advocates can secure legitimacy, then this is inevitably wrapped up in interrelationships with other personnel who more readily claim professional status. The idea of mental health advocacy is not new and arguably predates the advent of mental health services or professional psychiatric disciplines (Campbell 2001). To some extent, the resolution of perceived problems in the relationship between care teams and independent advocacy services is part of a wider project to ensure the very legitimacy of advocacy, in its many forms, is accepted within psychiatric services and wider society:

> Workers socialised into the power and false charity of
> medicalised models of care are similarly socialised into

dominated power relationships with clients which are dependent on the client remaining within the crushing, stultifying confines of the mental patient role. When an advocacy/empowerment practice asserts the oppression in that role, the fight for competing legitimacies erupts at every level. (Rose and Black 1985, pp.188–189)

Attacks by care providers on the legitimacy of independent advocacy have always been somewhat contradictory, given the remarked-upon evangelical espousal of an advocacy role amongst professional groups such as nurses and social workers (Dalrymple and Boylan 2013). Noting this state of affairs, David Brandon (1998, p.139) was able to ironically declaim: 'The function which was once despised and resisted, within a decade, becomes valuable enough to fight over!'

For some, this battle for legitimation is part of a much broader set of epistemic justice struggles, which ultimately aim to turn the tables and challenge the legitimacy of psychiatry itself (Fricker 2007; Radden 2012; Russo and Beresford 2014). Critically engaged practitioners and academics might support such political goals, possibly as part of the aforementioned radical professional and collective advocacy movements. In turn, this could tie in with service-level developments towards adoption of recovery approaches or alternative forms of care and treatment to simple bio-psychiatry. If services are to be demonstrably genuine in their commitment to recovery, then forms of independent advocacy that 'dictate neither the end nor the means' must perform a pivotal role (Stylianos and Kehyayan 2012, p.118).

Conclusions

Implicit to advocacy's social justice mechanism is a commitment to challenge inequality in its broadest sense. This involves challenging inequalities in mental health services and making sure that advocacy services themselves are as equitable as they can be so that everyone has the opportunity to have their rights promoted and defended. Yet, for Campbell (2009: 51), it is equally the case that 'now a right to advocacy has been partly recognized...service user influence over its provision is diminishing. In many respects, it is a choice between viewing the glass as half empty or half full.'

From the half-full perspective, we might look forward to an interesting future for advocacy as the policy rhetoric urges for more participation and involvement, for instance in care decisions framed by notions of co-production. Yet, tantalisingly, there are also increasing grounds for a more pessimistic outlook, with apparent propensity in services deepening and strengthening aspects of social control, coercion and compulsion. There is a concomitant trend towards homogenisation of advocacy and concentration of funding such that in many areas now IMHA is the only show in town, with other forms such as generic advocacy, citizen advocacy and collective advocacy being squeezed out. This has also denuded opportunities for peers and volunteers to undertake the advocacy role, and represents a distinct professionalisation trajectory for advocates. In effect, developments surrounding the introduction of IMHA raise concerns about creating a two-tier service, monopolising available funding and choking support for other forms of advocacy. Consolidation of larger third-sector organisations as providers of advocacy also, as Campbell notes, risks squeezing out opportunities for user influence, let alone control over advocacy, and also perhaps limits options for flexible localism in addressing the needs of minorities. In the worst case scenario options for diverse, high-quality advocacy would be severely diminished. Thus, the question for service users and survivors might be less about the glass being half full or half empty but, rather, whether the contents were what they asked for in the first place. In this sense, an increasingly uniform advocacy landscape could all end in 'tiers'.

Ultimately, legitimacy is framed by understandings of power relations. Interestingly, the survivor movement-inspired practices of advocacy and alternatives to bio-psychiatry also have supporters amongst the wider mental health care workforce. This opens up the possibility for progressive alliances seeking reform or even transformation of the system. Whilst we would concur with Sedgwick (1982) (see also Cresswell and Spandler 2009) that wholesale care for people in mental distress will always be necessary, and that this should at the very least be organised and funded by the state, the form that this takes need not be restricted by contemporary orthodoxy. Future mental health care could then begin to resemble or move beyond Campbell's (2009) glass half-full scenario. This would represent a much rosier prospect for independent advocacy indeed.

A4A Action For Advocacy

AIMS Accreditation for Inpatient Mental Health Services

AMHP Approved Mental Health Professional Replaced the Approved Social Worker role by the MH ACT 2007 and is responsible for organising and coordinating assessments under the MH Act.

BAME Black, Asian and Minority Ethnic

Best interests This usually refers to advocating or making decisions on someone else's behalf when they lack the capacity to do so for themselves.

DOLS (Deprivation of Liberty Safeguards) Safeguards for people deprived of their liberty but not covered by the MH Act 1983 safeguards.

Equality analysis Equality analysis is a way of considering the effect on different groups protected from discrimination by the Equality Act 2010.

IMCA (independent mental capacity advocate) A statutory advocate introduced by the MC Act 2005 to safeguard the interests of people lacking capacity.

Nearest relative This term is used in the MH Act 1983 to define someone who has certain rights and responsibilities to someone detained under the Act.

Non-instructed advocacy Non-instructed advocacy takes place when the person is unable to instruct or tell the person what they want.

Qualifying patients This refers to people who are detained under the MH Act who are eligible to use IMHA services.

Reasonable adjustments The Equality Act 2010 requires that reasonable adjustments should be made by public services to enable disabled people, including people with mental health conditions, to get the same standard of service as non-disabled people.

Safeguarding This refers to measures that can be taken to protect children and adults and who are vulnerable, as required by the Safeguarding Vulnerable Groups Act 2006.

Section 2 Admission under the MH Act 1983 for assessment for a maximum of 28 days.

Section 3 Admission under the MH Act 1983 for a treatment for up to six months, renewable for a further six months and then one year at a time.

Section 4 Admission under the MH Act 1983 in cases of emergency for a maximum of 72 hours.

Section 5 Compulsory detention of informal patients already in hospital for a maximum of 72 hours by an approved clinician or up to six hours by a suitably qualified nurse.

Section 57 Provisions relating to specific treatments such as psychosurgery, requiring individual consent, confirmation that the consent is valid and a second medical opinion.

Section 58 Provisions relating to specific treatments, such as extension of medication beyond three months or electro-convulsive therapy (ECT), requiring a second opinion appointed doctor (SOAD).

Tribunals The Tribunal is an independent judicial body that operates under the provisions of the MH Act 1983 (as amended by the MH Act 2007). Its main purpose is to review the cases of patients detained under the MH Act and to direct the discharge of any patients where the statutory criteria for detention are not met.

TUPE Transfer of Undertakings Protection of Employment Regulations 2006 protect employees' terms and conditions when a business goes through a transfer or takeover.

References

Legislation

International

European Convention on Human Rights (ECHR). Available at www.echr.coe.int/Documents/Convention_ENG.pdf, accessed on 9 April 2015.

United Nations Convention on the Rights of the Child. Available at www.unicef.org/gambia/UNCRC.pdf, accessed on 9 April 2015.

United Nations Convention on the Rights of Persons with Disabilities. Available at www.unicef.org.uk/Documents/Publication-pdfs/UNCRC_summary.pdf, accessed on 9 April 2015.

United Nations Declaration of Human Rights. Available at www.un.org/en/documents/udhr, accessed on 9 April 2015.

England and Wales

Care Act 2014. Available at www.legislation.gov.uk/ukpga/2014/23/contents/enacted, accessed on 9 April 2015.

Deprivation of Liberty Safeguards (DOLS) 2007. Available at http://webarchive.nationalarchives.gov.uk/+/www.dh.gov.uk/en/SocialCare/Deliveringadultsocialcare/MentalCapacity/MentalCapacityActDeprivationofLibertySafeguards/index.htm, accessed on 9 April 2015.

Equality Act 2010. Available at www.legislation.gov.uk/ukpga/2010/15, accessed on 9 April 2015.

Health and Social Care (Community Health and Standards) Act 2003. Available at www.legislation.gov.uk/ukpga/2003/43/contents, accessed on 9 April 2015.

Human Rights Act 1998. Available at www.legislation.gov.uk/ukpga/1998/42, accessed on 9 April 2015.

Mental Capacity Act 2005. Available at www.legislation.gov.uk/ukpga/2005/9/contents, accessed on 9 April 2015.

Mental Health Act 1983. Available at www.legislation.gov.uk/ukpga/1983/20/contents, accessed on 9 April 2015.

Mental Health (Amendment) Act 2007. Available at www.legislation.gov.uk/ukpga/2007/12/contents, accessed on 9 April 2015.

Public Sector Equality Duty (PSED). Available at www.gov.uk/equality-act-2010-guidance#public-sector-equality-duty, accessed on 9 April 2015.

11 Million and Young Minds (2008) *Out of the Shadows: A Review of the Response to Pushed into the Shadows: Young People's Experiences of Adult Mental Health Facilities.* London: 11 Million. Available at www.childrenscommissioner.gov.uk/content/publications/content_206, accessed on 11 November 2014.

Action for Advocacy (2006) *Quality Standards and Code of Practice for Advocacy Schemes.* London: Action for Advocacy.

Action for Advocacy (2008) *Here for Good? A Snapshot of the Advocacy Workforce.* London: Action for Advocacy.

Action for Advocacy (2009) *Lost in Translation: Outcomes of Advocacy Services.* Available at www.aqvx59.dsl.pipex.com/Lost_in_translation.pdf, accessed on 17 January 2015.

Action for Advocacy (2011) *Advocacy in a Cold Climate.* London: Action for Advocacy.

Action for Advocacy (2012) *IMHA Support Project: Key Competencies of an Effective IMHA Service.* London: Action for Advocacy.

Administrative Justice and Tribunals Council and Care Quality Commission (2011) *Patients' Experiences of the First-Tier Tribunal (Mental Health): Report of a Joint Pilot Project of the Administrative Justice and Tribunals Council and the Care Quality Commission.* Available at http://ajtc.justice.gov.uk/docs/AJTC__CQC_ First_tier_Tribunal_report_FINAL.pdf, accessed on 29 March 2015.

Ahern, K. and McDonald, S. (2002) 'The beliefs of nurses who were involved in a whistleblowing event.' *Journal of Advanced Nursing 38,* 303–309.

Aldridge, M. (2012) 'Addressing non adherence to antipsychotic medication: a harm-reduction approach.' *Journal of Psychiatric and Mental Health Nursing 19,* 85–96.

Allen, H. (1986) 'Psychiatry and the Construction of the Feminine.' In P. Miller and N. Rose (eds) *The Power of Psychiatry.* Cambridge: Polity Press.

AMICUS-MHNA, BAOT, BPS, COT, RCN and UNISON (2007) Press release: *Health Groups Suspend Membership of Mental Health Alliance.* Available at www.rcn.org. uk/newsevents/press_releases/uk/article2428, accessed on 29 March 2015.

Anderson, A. (2005) 'An introduction to theory of change.' *The Evaluation Exchange XI,* 2, 12–19.

Andreasson, E. and Skärsäter, I. (2012) 'Patients treated for psychosis and their perceptions of care in compulsory treatment: basis for an action plan.' *Journal of Psychiatric and Mental Health Nursing 19,* 1, 15–22.

Anthony, W.A. (1993) 'Recovery from mental illness: the guiding vision of the mental health service system in the 1990s.' *Psychiatric Rehabilitation Journal 16,* 4, 11–23.

Ashmore, R. and Banks, D. (2004) 'Student nurses' use of their interpersonal skills within clinical role-plays.' *Nurse Education Today 24,* 1, 20–29.

Askey, R., Holmshaw, J., Gamble, C. and Gray, R. (2009) 'What do carers of people with psychosis need from mental health services? Exploring the views of carers, service users and professionals.' *Journal of Family Therapy 31,* 3, 310–331.

Atkinson, J.M., Lorgelly, P., Reilly, J. and Stewart, A. (2007) *The Early Impact of the Administration of New Compulsory Powers Under the Mental Health (Care and Treatment) (Scotland) Act 2003.* Available at www.scotland.gov.uk/Publications, accessed on 20 January 2015.

Baker, P. (1989) *Hearing Voices.* A review of the work of Marius Romme and Sondra Escher of the Department of Social Psychiatry, Limburg University and the Community Health Centre, Maastricht. 2. Interview with Professor Marius Romme conducted by Paul Baker in November 1988. Manchester Alliance for Community Care/Manchester Mind/Salford Network/Trieste Fund.

Bamber, C. (2007) 'Listening to Patients in "Ashworth Time".' In D. Pilgrim (ed.) *Inside Ashworth: Professional Reflections of Institutional Life.* Oxford: Radcliffe Publishing.

Banks, C. and Redley, M. (2009) 'IMCAs in Their Second Year: The Experience of Key Stakeholders 2009. Appendix 2.' In Department of Health, *The Second Year of the Independent Mental Capacity Advocacy Service 2008/9.* London: Department of Health.

Banks, S. and Gallagher, A. (2009) *Ethics in Professional Life: Virtues for Health and Social Care.* Basingstoke: Palgrave Macmillan.

Barker, I., Newbigging, K. and Peck, E. (1997) 'Characteristics for sustained advocacy projects in mental health services.' *Journal of Integrated Care 5*, 4, 132–138.

Barker, I. and Peck, E. (1987) *Power in Strange Places.* London: Good Practices in Mental Health.

Barnes, D., Brandon, T. and Webb, T. (2002) *Independent Specialist Advocacy in England and Wales: Recommendations for Good Practice.* Durham: University of Durham.

Barnes, D. and Tate, A. (2000) *Advocacy from the Outside Inside: A Review of the Patients' Advocacy Service at Ashworth Hospital.* Durham: University of Durham/Ashworth Hospital Authority/North West Region NHS Secure Commissioning Team.

Barnes, M. (2007) *A Final Brick in the Wall? A History of the Nottingham Advocacy Group.* Available at http://eprints.brighton.ac.uk/10655, accessed on 17 January 2015.

Barnes, M. and Bowl, R. (2001) *Taking Over the Asylum: Empowerment and Mental Health.* Basingstoke: Palgrave Macmillan.

Barnes, M., Bowl, R. and Fisher, M. (1990) *Sectioned: Social Services and the Mental Health Act 1983.* London: Routledge.

Barnes, M. and Cotterell, P. (2012) 'Introduction: From Margin to Mainstream.' In M. Barnes and P. Cotterell (eds) *Critical Perspectives on User Involvement.* Bristol: Policy Press.

Barnes, M. and Gell, C. (2012) 'The Nottingham Advocacy Group: A Short History.' In M. Barnes and P. Cotterell (eds) *Critical Perspectives on User Involvement.* Bristol: Policy Press.

Basaglia, F. (1964) *The Destruction of the Mental Hospital as a Place of Institutionalisation: Thoughts Caused by Personal Experience with the Open Door System and Part Time Service.* London: First International Congress of Social Psychiatry.

Bateman, N. (1995) *Advocacy Skills for Health and Social Care Professionals.* Aldershot: Arena.

Bateman, N. (2000) *Advocacy Skills for Health and Social Care Professionals*, 2nd edition. London: Jessica Kingsley Publishers.

Bauer, A., Wistow, G., Dixon, J. and Knapp, M. (2013) *Investing in Advocacy Interventions for Parents with Learning Disabilities: What is the Economic Argument? Discussion Paper, 2860.* Kent: Personal Social Services Research Unit.

Beauchamp, T.L. (2007) 'The "Four Principles" Approach to Health Care Ethics.' In R. Ashcroft, A. Dawson, H. Draper and J. McMillan (eds) *Principles of Health Care Ethics.* Chichester: Wiley and Sons.

Beeforth, M., Conlan, E., Field, V., Hoser, B. and Sayce, L. (eds) (1990) *Whose Service is it Anyway? Users' Views on Co-ordinating Community Care.* London: RDP.

Bengtsson-Tops, A. and Svensson, B. (2010) 'Mental health users' experiences of being interviewed by another user in a research project: a qualitative study.' *Journal of Mental Health 19*, 3, 234–242.

Benjamin, E. (2011) 'Humanistic psychology and the mental health worker.' *Journal of Humanistic Psychology 51*, 1, 82–111.

Bentall, R. (2009) *Doctoring the Mind: Why Psychiatric Treatments Fail.* London: Allen Lane.

Bentall, R. (2013) 'Would a rose, by any other name, smell sweeter?' *Psychological Medicine 43*, 7, 1560–1562.

Beresford, P. (2002a) 'User involvement in research and evaluation: liberation or regulation?' *Social Policy and Society 1*, 2, 95–105.

Beresford, P. (2002b) 'Thinking about "mental health": towards a social model.' *Journal of Mental Health 11*, 581–584.

Beresford, P. (2005) 'Developing Self-Defined Social Approaches to Distress.' In S. Ramon and J. Williams (eds) *Mental Health at the Crossroads: The Promise of the Psychosocial Approach*. London: Ashgate.

Beresford, P., Nettle, M. and Perring, R. (2010) *Towards a Social Model of Madness and Distress: Exploring What Service Users Say*. York: Joseph Rowntree Foundation.

Berg-Cross, L., Reviere, R., Miller, J., Chappell, A. and Malmon, A. (2011) 'Certification of advocacy: a call to arms.' *Journal of Rural Psychology E14*, 1. Available at www.marshall.edu/jrcp/VE%2014%20N%201/JRCP%20Berg%20Cross%2014.1%20ready.pdf, accessed on 28 January 2015.

Bindman, J., Maingay, S. and Szmukler, G. (2003) 'The Human Rights Act and mental health legislation.' *British Journal of Psychiatry 182*, 91–94.

Blank, L., Peters, J., Pickvance, S., Wilford, J. and Macdonald, E. (2008) 'A systematic review of the factors which predict return to work for people suffering episodes of poor mental health.' *Journal of Occupational Rehabilitation 18*, 1, 27–34.

Bluglass, R. (1984) 'The origins of the Mental Health Act 1983: doctors in the house.' *Psychiatric Bulletin 8*, 7, 127–134.

Bola, J.R. and Mosher, L.R. (2003) 'Treatment of acute psychosis without neuroleptics: two-year outcomes from the Soteria project.' *The Journal of Nervous and Mental Disease 191*, 4, 219–229.

Bovaird, T., Dickinson, H. and Allen, K. (2012) *Commissioning Across Government: Review of Evidence*. Birmingham: Third Sector Research Centre, University of Birmingham.

Bowes, A. and Sim, D. (2006) 'Advocacy for Black and minority ethnic communities: understandings and expectations.' *British Journal of Social Work 36*, 7, 1209–1225.

Bracken, P. and Thomas, P. (2001) 'Postpsychiatry: a new direction for mental health.' *British Medical Journal 322*, 7288, 724–727.

Bracken, P. and Thomas, P. (2005) *Post-Psychiatry: Mental Health in a Post-Modern World*. Oxford: Oxford University Press.

Bracken, P., Thomas, P., Timimi, S., Asen, E. *et al.* (2012) 'Psychiatry beyond the current paradigm.' *British Journal of Psychiatry 201*, 430–434.

Bradley, A. (2008) *Non Instructed Advocacy Approaches*. POhWER. Internet Resource. Available at www.gain.org.uk/documents/Noninstructeedadvocacy.doc, accessed on 18 January 2015.

Brady, L. (2011) *Where is My Advocate? A Scoping Report on Advocacy Services for Children and Young People in England*. London: Office of the Children's Commissioner.

Brandon, D. (1998) 'Mental Health Advocacy.' In Y. Craig (ed.) *Advocacy, Counselling and Mediation in Casework*. London: Jessica Kingsley Publishers.

Brandon, D., Brandon, A. and Brandon, T. (1995) *Advocacy: Power to People with Disabilities*. Birmingham: Venture.

Brandon, D. and Brandon, T. (2000) 'The history of advocacy in mental health.' *Mental Health Practice 3*, 6, 6–8.

Breggin, P.R. (1991) *Toxic Psychiatry*. New York: St Martin's Press.

Brett, J., Staniszewska, S., Mockford, C., Herron-Marx, S. *et al.* (2014) 'Mapping the impact of patient and public involvement on health and social care research: a systematic review.' *Health Expectations 17*, 5, 637–650.

Broadbridge, A. (2012) *Developing Personalised Advocacy Outcomes: Learning from a Local Pilot Study*. Gateshead: Gateshead Advocacy Information Network.

Broadbridge, A. (2014) Personal communication.

Brooke, J. (2002) *Good Practice in Citizen Advocacy: Guidelines on Good Practice in Citizen Advocacy; Case Studies of Affiliation Among Advocacy Groups; Guidelines for Recognition of Citizen Advocates*. Glasgow: BILD Publications.

Brown, G., Standen, N. and Khilji, K. (2013) *Dementia Advocacy in a Time of Austerity.* Coventry: Coventry University. Available at www.opaal.org.uk/Libraries/ Local/1013/Docs/Dementia%20Advocacy%20in%20a%20time%20of%20 Austerity.pdf, accessed on 18 January 2014.

Bullmore, E., Fletcher, P. and Jones, P.B. (2009) 'Why psychiatry can't afford to be neurophobic.' *British Journal of Psychiatry 194,* 4, 293–295.

Burstow, B. and LeFrancois, B. (2014) 'Impassioned Praxis: An Introduction to Theorizing Resistance to Psychiatry.' In B. Burstow, B. LeFrancois and S.L. Diamond (eds) *Psychiatry Disrupted: Theorizing Resistance and Crafting the (R)Evolution.* Montreal, QC: McGill/Queen's University Press.

Burstow, B., LeFrancois, B. and Diamond, S.L. (eds) (2014) *Psychiatry Disrupted: Theorizing Resistance and Crafting the (R)Evolution.* Montreal, QC: McGill/Queen's University Press.

Busfield, J. (1996) *Men, Women and Madness: Understanding Gender and Mental Disorder.* London: Macmillan.

Butters, A., Webster, M. and Hill, M. (2010) *Understanding the Needs of People with Mental Health Conditions and/or Learning Disabilities and the Implications for the Pension, Disability and Carers Service.* London: DWP Publications.

Cabinet Office (2013) *The Commissioning Academy. Framework Document – An Introduction to Commissioning.* Available at www.gov.uk/government/publications/ the-commissioning-academy-framework-document, accessed on 18 January 2015.

Caldon, L.J.M., Marshall-Cork, H., Speed, G., Reed, M.W.R. and Collins, K.A. (2010) 'Consumers as researchers – innovative experiences in UK National Health Service research: consumers as researchers.' *International Journal of Consumer Studies 34,* 5, 547–550.

Calton, T., Ferriter, M., Huband, N. and Spandler, H. (2008) 'A systematic review of the Soteria paradigm for the treatment of people diagnosed with schizophrenia.' *Schizophrenia Bulletin 34,* 181–92.

Campbell, P. (1989) 'The Self-Advocacy Movement in the UK.' In A. Brackx and C. Grimshaw (eds) *Mental Health Care in Crisis.* London: Pluto.

Campbell, P. (1996) 'The History of the User Movement in the United Kingdom.' In T. Heller, J. Reynolds, R. Gomm, R. Muston et al. (eds) *Mental Health Matters: A Reader.* Basingstoke: Palgrave.

Campbell, P. (2001) 'From petitions to professionals.' *OpenMind 107,* 7.

Campbell, P. (2005) 'From Little Acorns – The Mental Health Service User Movement.' In A. Bell and P. Lindley (eds) *Beyond the Water Towers: The Unfinished Revolution in Mental Health Services 1985–2005.* London: Sainsbury Centre for Mental Health.

Campbell, P. (2009) 'The Service User/ Survivor Movement.' In J. Reynolds, R. Muston, T. Heller, J. Leach *et al.* (eds) *Mental Health Still Matters.* Basingstoke/Milton Keynes: Palgrave Macmillan/Open University Press.

Campbell, P. and Lindow, V. (1997) *Changing Practice: Mental Health Nursing and User Empowerment.* London: Mind and Royal College of Nursing.

Campbell, T. and Heginbotham, C. (1991) *Mental Illness: Prejudice, Discrimination and the Law.* Aldershot: Dartmouth.

Canvin, K., Bartlett, A. and Pinfold, V. (2002) 'A "bittersweet pill to swallow": learning from mental health service users' responses to compulsory community care in England.' *Health and Social Care in the Community 10,* 5, 361–369.

Carel, H. and Kidd, I.J. (2014) 'Epistemic injustice in healthcare: a philosophical analysis.' *Medicine, Health Care and Philosophy 17,* 529–540.

Carers Trust (2014) 'About Us.' *Carers Trust.* Available at www.carers.org/about, accessed on 30 June 2015.

Carlsson, H. (2014) 'Advocacy Changed My Life': Research into the Impact of Independent Advocacy on the Lives of People Experiencing Mental Illness. Edinburgh: SIAA.

Carpenter, M. (2009) 'A third wave, not a third way? New Labour, human rights and mental health in historical context.' Social Policy and Society 8, 2, 215–230.

Carr, S. (2014) Social Care for Marginalised Communities: Balancing Self-Organisation, Micro-Provision and Mainstream Support. London: Health Services Management Centre.

Carver, N. and Morrison, J. (2005) 'Advocacy in practice: the experiences of independent advocates on UK mental health wards.' Journal of Psychiatric and Mental Health Nursing 12, 1, 75–84.

Centre for Social Justice (2011) Completing the Revolution: Transforming Mental Health and Tackling Poverty. Available at www.centreforsocialjustice.org.uk/UserStorage/pdf/Pdf%20reports/CompletingtheRevolution.pdf, accessed on 18 January 2015.

Chamberlin, J. (1978) On Our Own: Patient-Controlled Alternatives to the Mental Health System. New York: Haworth Press.

Chamberlin, J. (1990) 'The ex-patients' movement: where we've been and where we're going.' Journal of Mind and Behavior 11, 3, 323–336.

Chamberlin, J. (1998) 'Citizenship rights and psychiatric disability.' Psychiatric Rehabilitation Journal 21, 4, 405.

Chamberlin, J. and Unzicker, R. (1990) Psychiatric Survivors, Ex-Patients, and Users: An Observation of Organisations in Holland and England. Unpublished manuscript.

Chase, E. (2008) 'Challenges and Complexities of Widening Access to Advocacy Services: Lessons from an Evaluation of Voice Advocacy Service.' In C.M. Oliver and J. Dalrymple (eds). Developing Advocacy for Children and Young People. London: Jessica Kingsley Publishers.

Chesler, P. (1974) Women and Madness. London: Allen Lane.

Children's Commissioner for England (2007) Pushed into the Shadows: Young People's Experience of Adult Mental Health Facilities. Office of the Children's Commissioner. Available at www.childrenscommissioner.gov.uk/content/publications/content_167, accessed on 25 January 2015.

Cleary, M. (2004) 'The realities of mental health nursing in acute inpatient environments.' International Journal of Mental Health Nursing 13, 53–60.

Cohen, D. and McCubbin, M. (1990) 'The political economy of tardive dyskinesia. Asymmetries in power and responsibility: challenging the therapeutic state.' Critical Perspectives on Psychiatry and the Mental Health System 11, 3, 3.

Coleman, C. and Dunmur, J. (2001) Surveying Mental Health Advocacy Needs in Sheffield. Sheffield: Sheffield Community Health Council.

Collins, S. (2009) 'Some critical perspectives on social work and collectives.' British Journal of Social Work 39, 2, 334–352.

Conlan, E. and Day, T. (eds) (1994) Advocacy – A Code of Practice. London: Department of Health.

Cooke, A. (ed.) (2014) Understanding Psychosis and Schizophrenia: Report for the British Psychological Society/Division of Clinical Psychology. London: BPS.

Cooke, B. and Kothari, U. (2002) Participation the New Tyranny? London: Zed Books.

CQC (Care Quality Commission) (2010) Mental Health Act Annual Report 2009/10. Available at www.cqc.org.uk/sites/default/files/documents/cqc_monitoring_the_use_of_the_mental_health_act_in_200910_main_report_tagged.pdf accessed on 5 June 2015.

CQC (Care Quality Commission) (2011) *Count Me In 2010: Results of the 2010 National Census of Inpatients and Patients on Supervised Community Treatment in Mental Health and Learning Disability Services in England and Wales.* London: CQC. Available at www.cqc.org.uk/sites/default/files/documents/count_me_in_2010_final_tagged.pdf accessed on 5 June 2015.

CQC (Care Quality Commission) (2012) *Mental Health Act Annual Report 2011/12.* Newcastle: CQC.

CQC (Care Quality Commission) (2013) *Mental Health Act Annual Report 2012/13.* Newcastle: CQC.

CQC (Care Quality Commission) (2014) *Monitoring the Mental Health Act in 2012/13.* Newcastle: CQC.

CQC (Care Quality Commission) (2015) *Monitoring the Mental Health Act in 2013/14.* Newcastle: CQC. Available at www.cqc.org.uk/sites/default/files/monitoring_the_mha_2013-14_report_web_0303.pdf.pdf, accessed on 8 March 2015.

CQC (Care Quality Commission) (2015b). Right here, Right now: People's experiences of help, care and support during a mental health crisis. Newcastle: CQC. Available at: http://www.cqc.org.uk/sites/default/files/20150611_CQC%20mhcrisis%20care%20report_FINAL_web.pdf, accessed on 30 June 2015.

Craig, G. (2013) 'Invisibilizing "race" in public policy.' *Critical Social Policy 33*, 4, 712–720.

Craig, Y. (1998) 'Conclusion.' In Y. Craig (ed.) *Advocacy, Counselling and Mediation in Casework.* London: Jessica Kingsley Publishers.

Craig, Y. and De Souza, M. (1998) 'Healthcare Decision Making and Mediation.' In Y. Craig (ed.) *Advocacy, Counselling and Mediation in Casework.* London: Jessica Kingsley Publishers.

Cresswell, M. (2009) 'Psychiatric survivors and experiential rights.' *Social Policy and Society 8*, 2, 231–243.

Cresswell, M. and Spandler, H. (2009) 'Psychopolitics: Peter Sedgwick's legacy for the politics of mental health.' *Social Theory and Health 7*, 2, 129–147.

Cresswell, M. and Spandler, H. (2013) 'The engaged academic: academic intellectuals and the psychiatric survivor movement.' *Social Movement Studies 12*, 2, 138–154.

Cromby, J. and Bell, V. (2015) 'Understandings of mental illness – mired in the past? Are psychological conceptions stuck in the 20th century?' *The Psychologist 28*, 1, 34–37.

Crossley, N. (2006) *Contesting Psychiatry: Social Movements in Mental Health.* Abingdon: Psychology Press.

Crowe, M. (2000) 'Constructing normality: a discourse analysis of the DSM-IV.' *Journal of Psychiatric and Mental Health Nursing 7*, 69–77.

Dalrymple, J. and Boylan, J. (2013) *Effective Advocacy in Social Work.* London: Sage Publications.

Davidson, L., Bellamy, C., Guy, K. and Miller, R. (2012) 'Peer support among persons with severe mental illnesses: a review of evidence and experience.' *World Psychiatry 11*, 2, 123–128.

Davies, C. (1995) *Gender and the Professional Predicament in Nursing.* Buckingham: Open University Press.

Davis, A. (2009) *Advocacy in Birmingham for People with Mental Health Issues.* Unpublished report.

Deegan, P. (1994) 'Recovery: The Lived Experience of Rehabilitation.' In W. Anthony and L. Spandiol (eds) *Readings in Psychiatric Rehabilitation.* Boston: Center for Psychiatric Rehabilitation.

Dementia Advocacy Network (2013) *Mind the Gap. Mapping London's Dementia Advocacy Services: A Report.* London: Dementia Advocacy Network.

Department of Health (1998) *Modernising Mental Health Services: Safe, Sound and Supportive*. London: Department of Health.

Department of Health (1999) *Report of the Expert Committee: Review of the Mental Health Act 1983*. London: Department of Health.

Department of Health (2003) *Mainstreaming Gender and Women's Mental Health: Implementation Guidance*. London: Department of Health.

Department of Health (2005a) *Government Response to the Report of the Joint Committee on the Draft Mental Health Bill 2004*. London: Department of Health. Available at www.gov.uk/government/uploads/system/uploads/attachment_data/file/272157/6624.pdf, accessed on 18 January 2015.

Department of Health (2005b) *Delivering Race Equality in Mental Health Care*. London: Department of Health.

Department of Health (2007) *Putting People First: A Shared Vision and Commitment to the Transformation of Adult Social Care*. Available at http://webarchive. nationalarchives.gov.uk/20130107105354/http:/www.dh.gov.uk/prod_consum_dh/groups/dh_digitalassets/@dh/@en/documents/digitalasset/dh_081119.pdf, accessed on 6 April 2015.

Department of Health (2008) *Standards: Appropriate Experience and Training*. Available at http://webarchive.nationalarchives.gov.uk/20130107105354/http://www.dh.gov.uk/prod_consum_dh/groups/dh_digitalassets/documents/digitalasset/dh_092056.pdf, accessed on 28 March 2015.

Department of Health (2009) *Independent Mental Health Advocates: Supplementary Guidance on Access to Patient Records Under Section 130B of the Mental Health Act 1983*. Available at www.dh.gov.uk/en/Publicationsandstatistics/publications/PublicationsPolicyAndGuidance/DH_098828, accessed on 14 January 2015.

Department of Health (2012) *Transforming Care: A National Response to Winterbourne View Hospital. Department of Health Review: Final Report*. London: Department of Health.

Department of Health (2013) *Post-Legislative Scrutiny of the Mental Health Act 2007: Response to the Report of the Health Committee of the House of Commons*. London: Department of Health.

Department of Health (2014a) *Requirements for Registration with the Care Quality Commission: Response to Consultations on Fundamental Standards, the Duty of Candour and the Fit and Proper Persons Requirement for Directors*. Available at www.gov.uk/government/consultations/fundamental-standards-for-health-and-social-care-providers, accessed on 15 January 2015.

Department of Health (2014b) *Consultation on Proposed Changes to the Mental Health Act 1983 Code of Practice*. Available at http://consultations.dh.gov.uk/mental-health-act-code-of-practice/consultation-on-proposed-changes-to-the-mental-hea/consult_view, accessed on 17 January 2015.

Department of Health (2015) *Mental Health 1983 Code of Practice*. Available at www.gov.uk/government/uploads/system/uploads/attachment_data/file/395494/mh-code.pdf, accessed on 15 January 2015.

Department of Health and Social Security (1980) *The Black Report. Inequalities in Health: Report of a Research Working Group*. London: The Stationery Office.

Donnison, D. (2009) *Speaking to Power: Advocacy for Health and Social Care*. Bristol: Policy Press.

Double, D. (2007) 'Adolf Meyer's psychobiology and the challenge for biomedicine.' *Philosophy, Psychiatry and Psychology 14*, 331–339.

Duxbury, J. (2011) 'Should nurses restrain violent and aggressive patients?' *Nursing Times 107*, 9, 22–25.

Duxbury, J. and Whittington, R. (2005) 'Causes and management of patient aggression and violence: staff and patient perspectives.' *Journal of Advanced Nursing 50*, 5, 469–478.

Eastman, N. (1994) 'Mental health law: civil liberties and the principle of reciprocity.' *British Medical Journal 308*, 6920, 43–45.

Equality and Human Rights Commission (2010) *Advocacy in Social Care for Groups Protected Under the Equality Legislation: Research Report 6.* Manchester: Equality and Human Rights Commission.

Etzioni, A. (1969) *The Semi-Professions and Their Organization.* New York: Free Press.

Evans-Lacko, S., Henderson, C. and Thornicroft, G. (2013) 'Public knowledge, attitudes and behaviour regarding people with mental illness in England 2009–2012.' *British Journal of Psychiatry 202*, 51–57.

Fanning, J. (2013) *Risk and the Mental Health Act 2007: Jeopardising Liberty, Facilitating Control?* Unpublished PhD thesis. Liverpool: University of Liverpool.

Fanning, J. (2014) *Risk and the Mental Health Act 2007: Jeopardising Liberty, Facilitating Control?* Seminar 9, October 2014, University of Birmingham Law School.

Fanon, F. (1952/2008) *Black Skin, White Masks.* New York: Grove Press.

Farquharson, C. (2014) *Launch of Commissioning for Better Outcomes at the National Children and Adult Services Conference.* Manchester, 30 October.

Faulkner, A. and Thomas, P. (2002) 'User-led research and evidence-based medicine.' *British Journal of Psychiatry 180*, 1, 1–3.

Fawcett, B. (2007) 'Consistencies and inconsistencies: mental health, compulsory treatment and community capacity building in England, Wales and Australia.' *British Journal of Social Work 37*, 6, 1027–1042.

Fazil, Q., Wallace, L., Singh, G., Ali, Z. and Bywaters, P. (2004) 'Empowerment and advocacy: reflections on action research with Bangladeshi and Pakistani families who have children with severe disabilities.' *Health and Social Care in the Community 12*, 5, 389–397.

Featherstone, B. and Fraser, C. (2012) 'I'm just a mother. I'm nothing special, they're all professionals: parental advocacy as an aid to parental engagement.' *Child and Family Social Work 17*, 2, 244–253.

Ferguson, I. and Lavalette, M. (2004) 'Beyond power discourse: alienation and social work.' *British Journal of Social Work 34*, 3, 297–312.

Ferguson, I. and Lavalette, M. (2006) 'Globalization and global justice: towards a social work of resistance.' *International Social Work 49*, 3, 309–318.

Finkelstein, V. (2007) *The 'Social Model of Disability' and the Disability Movement.* Manchester: Greater Manchester Coalition of Disabled People.

Fistein, E.C., Holland, A.J., Clare, I.C.H. and Gunn, M.J. (2009) 'A comparison of mental health legislation from diverse Commonwealth jurisdictions.' *International Journal of Law and Psychiatry 32*, 3, 147–155.

Fleischmann, P. (2014) Personal communication.

Foley, R. and Platzer, H. (2007) 'Place and provision: mapping mental health advocacy services in London.' *Social Science and Medicine 64*, 3, 617–632.

Foucault, M. (1965) *Madness and Civilization: A History of Insanity in the Age of Reason.* New York: Random House.

Foucault, M. (2003) *Abnormal: Lectures at the Collège De France 1974–1975.* New York: Picador.

Fourie, W., McDonald, S., Connor, J. and Bartlett, S. (2005) 'The role of the registered nurse in an acute mental health inpatient setting in New Zealand: perceptions versus reality.' *International Journal of Mental Health Nursing 14*, 134–141.

Francis, E., David, J., Johnson, N. and Sashidharan, S.P. (1989) 'Black people and psychiatry in the UK: an alternative to institutional care.' *Psychiatric Bulletin 13*, 9, 482–485.

Francis, R. (2013) *Report of the Mid Staffordshire NHS Foundation Trust Public Inquiry.* London: Stationery Office.

Fricker, M. (2007) *Epistemic Injustice: Power and the Ethics of Knowing.* Oxford: Oxford University Press.

Fromm, E. (1956) *The Sane Society.* London: Routledge and Kegan Paul.

Gamble, D. (1999) 'The value of advocacy: putting ethics in to practice.' *Psychiatric Bulletin 23*, 569–570.

Gault, I. (2009) 'Service user and carer perspectives on compliance and compulsory treatment in community mental health services.' *Health and Social Care in the Community 17*, 5, 504–513.

Gerson, R., Davidson, L., Booty, A., McGlashan, T. *et al.* (2009) 'Families' experience with seeking treatment for recent-onset psychosis.' *Psychiatric Services 60*, 6, 812–816.

Ghaemi, S.N. (2009) 'The rise and fall of the biopsychosocial model.' *British Journal of Psychiatry 195*, 3–4.

Gibbs, A., Dawson, J., Ansley, C. and Mullen, R. (2005) 'How patients in New Zealand view community treatment orders.' *Journal of Mental Health 14*, 4, 357–368.

Gilburt, H., Rose, D. and Slade, M. (2008) 'The importance of relationships in mental health care: a qualitative study of service users' experiences of psychiatric hospital admission in the UK.' *BMC Health Services Research 8*, 1, 92.

Gillard, S., Borschmann, R., Turner, K., Goodrich-Purnell, N., Lovell, K. and Chambers, M. (2010) '"What difference does it make?" Finding evidence of the impact of mental health service user researchers on research into the experiences of detained psychiatric patients: impact of mental health service user researchers on research.' *Health Expectations 13*, 2, 185–194.

Glasgow University Media Group (1996) *Media and Mental Distress.* Harlow: Addison-Wesley Longman.

Goffman, E. (1961) *Asylums: Essays on the Social Situation of Mental Patients and Other Inmates.* New York: Anchor Books.

Goffman, E. (1963) *Stigma: Notes on the Management of Spoiled Identity.* New York: Simon and Schuster.

Goodwin, S. (1997) 'Independence, risk and compulsion: conflicts in mental health policy.' *Social Policy and Administration 31*, 3, 260–273.

Goss, S. and Miller, C. (1995) *From Margin to Mainstream: Developing User and Carer Centred Community Care.* York: Joseph Rowntree Foundation.

Gostin, L.O. (2000) 'Human rights of persons with mental disabilities: the European Convention of Human Rights.' *International Journal of Law and Psychiatry 23*, 2, 125–159.

Gostin, L.O. (1990) 'The rights stuff.' *OpenMind 47*, 12–13.

Gostin, L.O. (2008) '"Old" and "new" institutions for persons with mental illness: treatment, punishment or preventive confinement?' *Public Health 122*, 9, 906–913.

Government Equalities Office (2012) *Public Sector Equality Duty.* Available at www.gov.uk/government/publications/public-sector-equality-duty, accessed on 10 April 2015.

Gray, J. (1985) 'Planning for Individuals.' In T. McAusland (ed.) *Planning and Monitoring Community Mental Health Centres.* London: King's Fund.

Gray, R., Wykes, T. and Gournay, K. (2002) 'From compliance to concordance: a review of the literature on interventions to enhance compliance with antipsychotic medication.' *Journal of Psychiatric and Mental Health Nursing 9*, 3, 277–284.

Gregory, M., Newbigging, K., Cole, A. and Pearsall, A. (2003) *Working Together: Developing and Providing Services for People with Learning Disabilities and Mental Health Problems*. London: Institute for Applied Health and Social Policy/Centre for Mental Health Services Development.

Grob, G.N. (2011) 'The attack of psychiatric legitimacy in the 1960s: rhetoric and reality.' *Journal of the History of the Behavioral Sciences 47*, 4, 398–416.

Haglund, K., von Knorring, L. and von Essen, L. (2003) 'Forced medication in psychiatric care: patient experiences and nurse perceptions.' *Journal of Psychiatric and Mental Health Nursing 10*, 1, 65–72.

Hakim, R. and Pollard, T. (2011) *Independent Mental Health Advocacy: Briefing Paper 3*. London: Mental Health Alliance. Available at www.mentalhealthalliance.org.uk/resources/Independent_Mental_Health_Advocacy_report.pdf, accessed on 18 January 2015.

Hall, W. (2012) *Harm Reduction Guide to Coming off Psychiatric Drugs*. New York: Icarus Project.

Hansard (2009) HC Mental health advocacy Deb, 12 January, vol 486, col 109.

Happell, B., Manias, E. and Pinikahana, J. (2002) 'The role of the inpatient mental health nurse in facilitating patient adherence to medication regimes.' *International Journal of Mental Health Nursing 11*, 251–259.

Harnett, R. (2004) 'Doing peer advocacy: insights from the field.' *Representing Children 17*, 2, 131–141.

Harper, D. and Speed, E. (2014) 'Uncovering Recovery: The Resistable Rise of Recovery and Resilience.' In E. Speed, J. Moncrieff and M. Rapley (eds) *De-Medicalizing Misery II: Society, Politics and the Mental Health Industry*. Basingstoke: Palgrave Macmillan.

Harrington, V. (2009) 'Innovation in a backwater: the Harpurhey Resettlement Team and the mental health services of North Manchester, 1982–1987.' *Health & Place 15*, 3, 664–671.

Harrison, T. and Davis, R. (2009) 'Advocacy: time to communicate.' *Advances in Psychiatric Treatment 15*, 57–64.

Health Services Management Centre (2014a) *Commissioning for Better Outcomes: A Literature Review*. Unpublished paper.

Health Services Management Centre (2014b) *Commissioning for Better Outcomes: A Route Map*. Birmingham: HSMC.

Heginbotham, C. (2012) *Values-Based Commissioning of Health and Social Care*. Cambridge: Cambridge University Press.

Henderson, C., Flood, C., Leese, M., Thornicroft, G., Sutherby, K. and Szmukler, G. (2004) 'Effect of joint crisis plans on use of compulsory treatment in psychiatry: single blind randomised controlled trial.' *British Medical Journal 329*, 136.

Henderson, C., Jackson, C., Slade, M., Young, A.S. and Strauss, J.L. (2010) 'How should we implement psychiatric advance directives? Views of consumers, caregivers, mental health providers and researchers.' *Administration and Policy in Mental Health and Mental Health Services Research 37*, 6, 447–458.

Henderson, R. and Pochin, M. (2001) *A Right Result? Advocacy, Justice and Empowerment*. Bristol: Policy Press.

Herlihy, D.P. and Holloway, F. (2009) 'The Mental Health Act and the Mental Capacity Act: untangling the relationship.' *Psychiatry 8*, 12, 478–480.

Hervey, N. (1986) 'Advocacy or folly: the alleged lunatics' friends society, 1845–63.' *Medical History 30*, 245–275.

Hiday, V.A., Swartz, M.S., Swanson, J. and Wagner, H.R. (1997) 'Patient perceptions of coercion in mental hospital admission.' *International Journal of Law and Psychiatry 20*, 2, 227–241.

Hoekstra, T., Lendemeijer, H. and Jansen, M. (2004) 'Seclusion: the inside story.' *Journal of Psychiatric and Mental Health Nursing 11*, 3, 276–283.

Holmes, D. (2001) 'From iron gaze to nursing care: mental health nursing in the era of panopticism.' *Journal of Psychiatric and Mental Health Nursing 8*, 7–15.

Hooff, S. and Goossensen, A. (2013) 'How to increase quality of care during coercive admission? A review of literature.' *Scandinavian Journal of Caring Sciences 28*, 425–434.

Hubinette, M., Dobson, S., Voyer, S. and Regehr, G. (2014) '"We" not "I": health advocacy is a team sport.' *Medical Education 48*, 9, 895–901.

Hughes, R., Hayward, M. and Finlay, W.M.L. (2009) 'Patients' perceptions of the impact of involuntary inpatient care on self, relationships and recovery.' *Journal of Mental Health 18*, 2, 152–160.

Hugman, R. (1991) *Power in Caring Professions*. Basingstoke: Macmillan.

Independent Advisory Panel on Deaths in Custody (2014) *Statistical Analysis of All Recorded Deaths of Individuals Detained in State Custody Between 1 January 2000 and 31 December 2012*. Available at http://iapdeathsincustody.independent.gov.uk/wp-content/uploads/2014/05/IAP-Statistical-analysis-of-recorded-deaths-2000-to-2012-Publication.pdf, accessed on 18 January 2015.

Ingleby, D. (1985) 'Professionals as socializers: the "psy complex".' *Research in Law, Deviance and Social Control 7*, 79, 109.

Ivers, V. (1994) *Citizen Advocacy in Action: Working with Older People*. Stoke on Trent: Beth Johnson Foundation.

Ivers, V. (1998) 'Advocacy.' In Y. Craig (ed.) *Advocacy, Counselling and Mediation in Casework*. London: Jessica Kingsley Publishers.

Jackson, D. (2008) 'Editorial: what becomes of the whistleblowers?' *Journal of Clinical Nursing 17*, 1261–1262.

James, A. (2010) 'A beacon of help.' *Mental Health Today*, February, 18–19.

Jankovic, J., Richards, F. and Priebe, S. (2010) 'Advance statements in adult mental health.' *Advances in Psychiatric Treatment 16*, 6, 448–455.

Jenny, J. (1979) 'Patient advocacy – another role for nursing.' *International Nursing Review 26*, 176–181.

Johansson, I.M. and Lundman, B. (2002) 'Patients' experience of involuntary psychiatric care: good opportunities and great losses.' *Journal of Psychiatric and Mental Health Nursing 9*, 6, 639–647.

Johnson, R. and Haigh, R. (2011) 'Social psychiatry and social policy for the 21st century: new concepts for new needs – the "Enabling Environments" initiative.' *Mental Health and Social Inclusion 15*, 1, 17–23.

Joint Committee on the Draft Mental Health Bill (2005) *Session 2004–2005. House of Lords, House of Commons, UK Parliament*. Available at www.publications.parliament.uk/pa/jt/jtment.htm, accessed on 18 January 2015.

Jones, C., Ferguson, I., Lavalette, M. and Penketh, L. (2004) *Social Work and Social Justice: A Manifesto for a New Engaged Practice*. Available at www.socialworkfuture.org/attachments/article/56/SWAN%20Social%20Work%20Manifesto.pdf, accessed on 18 January 2015.

Jonikas, J.A., Grey, D.D., Copeland, M.E., Razzano, L.A. et al. (2013) 'Improving propensity for patient self-advocacy through wellness recovery action planning: results of a randomized controlled trial.' *Community Mental Health Journal 49*, 3, 260–269.

Jugessur, T. and Iles, I. (2009) 'Advocacy in mental health nursing: an integrative review of the literature.' *Journal of Psychiatric and Mental Health Nursing 16*, 187–195.

Kalathil, J. (2011) *Dancing to Our Own Tunes: Reassessing Black and Minority Ethnic Service User Involvement. Reprint of the 2008 Report with a Review of Work to Take the Recommendations Forward.* London: The Afiya Trust and National Survivor User Network (NSUN). Available at www.nsun.org.uk/assets/downloadableFiles/dancing-to-our-own-tunes---report.pdf, accessed on 15 January 2015.

Kalathil, J. and Faulkner, A. (2015) 'Racialisation and knowledge production: a critique of the report "Understanding Psychosis and Schizophrenia".' *Mental Health Today*, Jan–Feb, 22–23.

Katsakou, C., Marougka, S., Garabette, J., Rost, F., Yeeles, K. and Priebe, S. (2011) 'Why do some voluntary patients feel coerced into hospitalisation? A mixed-methods study.' *Psychiatry Research 187*, 1, 275–282.

Katsakou, C. and Priebe, S. (2007) 'Patients' experiences of involuntary hospital admission and treatment: A review of qualitative studies.' *Epidemiologia E Psichiatria Sociale 16*, 2, 172–178.

Katsakou, C., Rose, D., Amos, T., Bowers, L., McCabe, R., Oliver, D. and Priebe, S. (2012) 'Psychiatric patients' views on why their involuntary hospitalisation was right or wrong: a qualitative study.' *Social Psychiatry and Psychiatric Epidemiology 47*, 7, 1169–1179.

Keating, F. (2007) *African and Caribbean Men and Mental Health: A Race Equality Foundation Briefing Paper.* Available at www.better-health.org.uk/sites/default/files/briefings/downloads/health-brief5.pdf, accessed on 18 January 2015.

Keating, F., Robertson, D., McCulloch, A. and Francis, E. (2002) *Breaking the Circles of Fear: A Review of the Relationship between Mental Health Services and African and Caribbean Communities.* London: Sainsbury Centre for Mental Health.

Kelly, B.D. (2011) 'Mental health legislation and human rights in England, Wales and the Republic of Ireland.' *International Journal of Law and Psychiatry 34*, 6, 439–454.

Kendell, R. (2001) 'The distinction between mental and physical illness.' *British Journal of Psychiatry 178*, 490–493.

Kendell, R. (1993) 'The Nature of Psychiatric Disorders.' In T. Heller, J. Reynolds, R. Gomm, R. Muston and S. Pattison (eds) *Mental Health Matters: A Reader.* Basingstoke: Macmillan in association with the Open University.

Khan, M. and Daw, R. (2011) *Do the Right Thing: How to Judge a Good Ward.* London: Royal College of Psychiatrists.

Kinderman, P., Read, J., Moncrieff, J. and Bentall, R.P. (2013) 'Drop the language of disorder.' *Evidence Based Mental Health 16*, 2–3.

Kontio, R., Joffe, G., Putkonen, H., Kuosmanen, L. *et al.* (2012) 'Seclusion and restraint in psychiatry: patients' experiences and practical suggestions on how to improve practices and use alternatives.' *Perspectives in Psychiatric Care 48*, 1, 16–24.

Lacey Y. and Thomas P. (2001) 'A survey of psychiatrists' and nurses' views of mental health advocacy.' *Psychiatric Bulletin 25*, 477–480.

Lafrance, M.N. and McKenzie-Mohr, S. (2013) 'The DSM and its lure of legitimacy.' *Feminism and Psychology 23*, 1, 119–140.

Laing, R.D. (1960) *The Divided Self.* London: Tavistock Publications.

Laing, R.D. (1967) *The Politics of Experience and the Bird of Paradise.* Harmondsworth: Penguin Books.

Lawton, A. (2006) *Supporting Self-Advocacy.* Stakeholder Position Paper 06. London: SCIE.

Lawton, A. (2009) *Personalisation and Learning Disabilities: A Review of Evidence on Advocacy and its Practice for People with Learning Disabilities and High Support Needs.* Adults' Services Paper 24. London: SCIE. Available at www.scie.org.uk/publications/reports/report24.pdf, accessed on 18 January 2015.

Layard, R. (2013) 'Mental health: the new frontier for labour economics.' *IZA Journal of Labor Policy 2,* 1, 1–16.

LeFrancois, B., Menzies, R. and Reaume, G. (eds) (2014) *Mad Matters: A Critical Reader in Canadian Mad Studies.* Toronto: Canadian Scholars Press.

Lepping, P. (2007) 'Ethical analysis of the new proposed mental health legislation in England and Wales.' *Philosophy, Ethics and Humanities 2,* 5.

Liegghio, M. (2013) 'A Denial of Being: Psychiatrization as Epistemic Violence.' In B. Lefrançois, R. Menzies and G. Reaume (eds) *Mad Matters: A Critical Reader in Canadian Mad Studies.* Toronto: Canadian Scholars Press.

Lindow, V. (1991) 'Experts, lies and stereotypes.' *Health Service Journal,* 29 August, 18.

Lipsky, M. (1980) *Street Level Bureaucracy: Dilemmas and the Individual in Public Services.* New York: Sage.

Luchins, D.J. (2004) 'At issue: will the term brain disease reduce stigma and promote parity for mental illnesses?' *Schizophrenia Bulletin 30,* 4, 1043–1048.

Lukes, S. (1974/2005) *Power: A Radical View.* London: Macmillan.

McCabe, J. (1996) 'Women in special hospitals and secure psychiatric containment.' *Mental Health Review Journal 1,* 2, 28–30.

McCommon, B. (2006) 'Antipsychiatry and the gay rights movement.' *Psychiatric Services 57,* 12, 1809.

McKeown, M. (2012a) 'William Neville Bingley: an appreciation.' *Asylum: The Magazine for Democratic Psychiatry 19,* 2, 6.

McKeown, M. (2012b) 'Advocating for advocacy. William's legacy in advocacy and involvement: research, education and practice.' *The William Bingley Memorial Symposium: Distress and Detention. Rethinking Mental Health Law.* Lancaster: University of Lancaster.

McKeown, M., Bingley, W. and Denoual, I. (2002) *A Review of Advocacy Services at the Edenfield Regional Secure Unit and Bowness High Dependency Unit, Prestwich Hospital.* Preston: UCLan/North West Secure Commissioning Team.

McKeown, M. and Jones, F. (2014) 'Service User Involvement.' In I. Hulatt (ed.) *Mental Health Policy for Nurses.* London: Sage.

McKeown, M., Malihi-Shoja, L., Downe, S. and The Comensus Writing Collective (2010) *Service User and Carer Involvement in Education for Health and Social Care.* Oxford: Wiley-Blackwell.

McKeown, M., Poursanidou, D., Able, L., Newbigging, K., Ridley, J. and Kiansumba, M. (2013) 'Independent mental health advocacy: still cooling out the mark?' *Mental Health Today,* November/December, 20–21.

McKeown, M., Ridley, J., Newbigging, K., Machin, K., Poursanidou, K. and Cruse, K. (2014a) 'Conflict of roles: A conflict of ideas? The unsettled relations between care team staff and independent mental health advocates.' *International Journal of Mental Health Nursing 23,* 5, 398–408.

McKeown, M., Cresswell, M. and Spandler, H. (2014b) 'Deeply Engaged Relationships: Alliances Between Mental Health Workers and Psychiatric Survivors in the UK.' In B. Burstow, B.A. LeFrancois and S.L. Diamond (eds) *Psychiatry Disrupted: Theorizing Resistance and Crafting the (R)Evolution.* Montreal, QC: McGill/Queen's University Press.

McKeown, M., Jones, F., Wright, K., Spandler, H. *et al.* (2014c) 'It's the talk: a study of involvement practices in secure mental health services.' *Health Expectations.* DOI: 10.111/hex.12232.

McKeown, M. and Stowell-Smith, M. (2006) 'The comforts of evil: dangerous personalities in high security hospitals and the horror film.' In T. Mason (ed.) *Forensic Psychiatry: The Influences of Evil.* Totowa, NJ: Humana Press.

McLaren, N. (1998) 'A critical review of the biopsychosocial model.' *The Australian and New Zealand Journal of Psychiatry 32,* 1, 86–92; discussion 93–96.

Mclean, C., Campbell, C. and Cornish, F. (2003) 'African-Caribbean interactions with mental health services in the UK: experiences and expectations of exclusion as (re) productive of health inequalities.' *Social Science & Medicine 56,* 3, 657–669.

Macadam, A., Watts, R. and Greig, R. (2013) *The Impact of Advocacy for People who Use Social Care Services: Scoping Review.* London: School for Social Care Research.

Mackler, D. (2014) *Healing Homes: An Alternative, Swedish Model for Healing Psychosis.* Film. Available at www.pccs-books.co.uk/products/healing-homes-an-alternative-swedish-model-for-healing-psychosis/#.VJgEToN8A, accessed on 18 January 2015.

Maden, A. (2007) 'England's new Mental Health Act represents law catching up with science: a commentary on Peter Lepping's ethical analysis of the new mental health legislation in England and Wales.' *Philosophy, Ethics and Humanities in Medicine 2,* 1, 16.

Mallik, M. (1997) 'Advocacy in nursing – a review of the literature.' *Journal of Advanced Nursing 25,* 130–138.

Marcuse, H. (1964) *One Dimensional Man.* London: Routledge and Kegan Paul.

Martin, P. and Mullins, G. (2008) *A Review of Advocacy in Suffolk.* Suffolk: Suffolk County Council.

Martins, C.D.S., Willner, P., Brown, A. and Jenkins, R. (2011) 'Knowledge of advocacy options within services for people with learning disabilities.' *Journal of Applied Research in Intellectual Disabilities 24,* 3, 274–279.

Masterson, S. and Owen, S. (2006) 'Mental health service users' social and individual empowerment: using theories of power to elucidate far-reaching strategies.' *Journal of Mental Health 15,* 1, 19–34.

Means, R., Richards, S. and Smith, R. (2008) *Community Care,* 4th edition. Basingstoke: Palgrave Macmillan.

Meehan, T., Bergen, H. and Fjeldsoe, K. (2004) 'Staff and patient perceptions of seclusion: has anything changed?' *Journal of Advanced Nursing 47,* 1, 33–38.

Mental Health Alliance (2005) *Towards a Better Mental Health Act: The Mental Health Alliance Policy Agenda.* Available at www.mentalhealthalliance.org.uk/pre2007/policyagenda.html, accessed on 18 January 2015.

Mental Health Alliance (2007) *The Mental Health Act 2007: A Final Report.* Available at www.mentalhealthalliance.org.uk/news/prfinalreport.html, accessed on 29 March 2015.

Mental Health Alliance (2008) *New Mental Health Powers Must Be Used Wisely, Says Alliance.* Available at www.mentalhealthalliance.org.uk/news/prpowersusedwisely.html, accessed on 18 January 2015.

Mental Health Recovery Study Working Group (2009) *Mental Health 'Recovery': Users and Refusers.* Toronto: Wellesley Institute.

Mercer, K. (1986) 'Racism and Transcultural Psychiatry.' In P. Miller and N. Rose (eds) *The Power of Psychiatry.* Cambridge: Polity Press.

Miller, B., Mansen, T. and Lee, H. (1983) 'Patient advocacy: do nurses have the power and authority to act as patient advocate?' *Nursing Leadership 6,* 56–60.

Miller, E. (2011) *Measuring Personal Outcomes: Challenges and Strategies. IRISS Insights No. 12.* Glasgow: Institute for Research and Innovation in Social Services. Available at www.iriss.org.uk/sites/default/files/iriss-insight-12.pdf, accessed on 18 January 2015.

Mind (1992) *The Mind Guide to Advocacy in Mental Health: Empowerment in Action.* London: Mind.

Mind (2006) *With us in Mind: Service User Recommendations for Advocacy Standards in England.* London: Mind.

Mind (2010) *Advocacy in Mental Health.* London: Mind. Available at www.Mind.org.uk/information-support/guides-to-support-and-services/advocacy-in-mental-health/#.VJamBoN8A, accessed on 18 January 2015.

Ministry of Justice (2011) *Practice Note: Role of the Independent Mental Health Advocate ('IMHA') in First-Tier Tribunal (Mental Health) Hearings.* Mental Health Law On-Line. Available at www.mentalhealthlaw.co.uk/Practice_Note:_Role_of_the_Independent_Mental_Health_Advocate_in_First-tier_Tribunal_(Mental_Health)_Hearings, accessed on 29 March 2015.

Mir, G. and Nocon, A. (2002) 'Partnerships, advocacy and independence.' *Journal of Learning Disabilities 6,* 2, 153–162.

Moncrieff, J. (2003a) *Is Psychiatry for Sale? An Examination of the Influence of the Pharmaceutical Industry on Academic and Practical Psychiatry.* Maudsley Discussion Paper No. 13. London: Institute of Psychiatry.

Moncrieff, J. (2003b) 'The politics of a new Mental Health Act.' *The British Journal of Psychiatry 183,* 8-9.

Moncrieff, J. (2006) 'Psychiatric drug promotion and the politics of neoliberalism.' *British Journal of Psychiatry 188,* 301–302.

Moncrieff, J. (2009) *The Myth of the Chemical Cure: A Critique of Psychiatric Drug Treatment.* Basingstoke: Palgrave Macmillan.

Moncrieff, J. (2013) *The Bitterest Pills: The Troubling Story of Antipsychotic Drugs.* Basingstoke: Palgrave Macmillan.

Morgan, C. (2012) 'Ethnicity and the long-term course and outcome of psychosis: initial findings from AESOP-10.' *Schizophrenia Research 136,* S42–S43.

Morrison, A.P., Turkington, D., Pyle, M., Spencer, H. *et al.* (2014) 'Cognitive therapy for people with schizophrenia spectrum disorders not taking antipsychotic drugs: a single-blind randomised controlled trial.' *The Lancet 383,* 9926, 1395–1403.

Morrison, L. (2005) *Talking Back to Psychiatry: The Psychiatric Consumer/Survivor/Ex-Patient Movement.* New York: Routledge.

Morse, S.J. (1982) 'A preference for liberty: the case against involuntary commitment of the mentally disordered.' *California Law Review 70,* 1, 54–106.

Mosher, L. (1999) 'Soteria and other alternatives to acute psychiatric hospitalization: a personal and professional review.' *Journal of Nervous and Mental Disease 187,* 142–149.

Mueser, K.T., Deavers, F., Penn, D.L. and Cassisi, J.E. (2013) 'Psychosocial treatments for schizophrenia.' *Annual Review of Clinical Psychology 9,* 465–497.

NDTi (National Development Team for inclusion) (2012) *Reasonably Adjusted? Mental Health Services for People with Autism and People with Learning Disabilities.* Available at www.ndti.org.uk/uploads/files/NHS_Confederation_report_Submitted_version.pdf, accessed on 9 April 2015.

National Health Service (NHS) Information Centre (2011) *Inpatients Formally Detained in Hospitals Under the Mental Health Act 1983 and Patients Subject to Supervised Community Treatment – England, 2010–2011, Annual Figures.* Available at www.hscic.gov.uk/pubs/inpatientdetmha1011, accessed on 26 January 2014.

National Mental Health Development Unit (2009a) *Independent Mental Health Advocacy: Effective Practice Guide.* London: NMHDU.

National Mental Health Development Unit (2009b) *Independent Mental Health Advocacy (Level 4): Workbook for Independent Study.* Available at http://webarchive. nationalarchives.gov.uk/20100304081458/http://www.nmhdu.org.uk/news/ shoulder-to-shoulder--a-new-dvd-for-imha, accessed on 18 January 2015.

National Mental Health Development Unit (2011) *Accessible Mental Health Services: Provision for Deaf People.* Available at http://webarchive.nationalarchives.gov. uk/20110512085250/www.nmhdu.org.uk/silo/files/accessible-mental-health-services.pdf, accessed on 18 January 2015.

National Voices and Think Local Act Personal (2014) *No Assumptions: a Narrative for Personalised, Coordinated Care and Support in Mental Health.* London: National Voices/Think Local Act Personal/NHS England.

Nelson, M. (1988) 'Advocacy in nursing.' *Nursing Outlook 36,* 136–141.

Newbigging, K. and McKeown, M. (2007) 'Mental health advocacy with Black and minority ethnic communities: conceptual and ethical implications.' *Current Opinion in Psychiatry 20,* 588–593.

Newbigging, K., Cadman, A. and Westley, J. (1989) 'Powell Street: Community Mental Health.' In D. Seedhouse and A. Cribb (eds) *Changing Ideas in Health Care.* Chichester: Wiley.

Newbigging, K., McKeown, M., Hunkins-Hutchinson, E.A., French, B. *et al.* (2007) *SCIE Knowledge Review 15. Mtetezi: Developing Mental Health Advocacy with African and Caribbean Men.* London: Social Care Institute for Excellence.

Newbigging, K., McKeown, M., Habte-Mariam, Z., Mullings, D., Charles, J.J. and Holt, K. (2008) *Commissioning and Providing Mental Health Advocacy for African and Caribbean Men: A Resource Guide.* Available at www.scie.org.uk/publications/ guides/guide21, accessed on 18 January 2015.

Newbigging, K., Paul, J., Waterhouse, S. and Freese, C. (2010) *Working Towards Women's Well-Being: Unfinished Business.* London: NMHDU.

Newbigging, K., Ridley, J., McKeown, M., Machin, K., Poursanidou, K. Able, L., Cruse, K., Grey, P., De la Haye, S., Habte-Mariam, Z., Joseph, D., Kiansumba, M. and Sadd, J. (2012a) *The Right to be Heard: Review of the Quality of IMHA Services. Report for the Department of Health.* Preston: University of Central Lancashire.

Newbigging, K., Roy, A., McKeown, M., French, B. and Habte-Mariam, Z. (2012b) 'Involving Ethnically Diverse Service Users in the Research Process: Alliances and Action.' In P. Beresford and S. Carr (eds) *Social Care, Service Users and User Involvement: Building on Research.* London: Jessica Kingsley Publishers.

Newbigging, K., Ridley, J., McKeown, M., Machin, K. and Poursanidou, K. (2014) '"When you haven't got much of a voice": an evaluation of the quality of independent mental health advocate (IMHA) services in England.' *Health and Social Care in the Community,* DOI: 10.1111/hsc.12153.

NICE (National Institute for Health and Care Excellence) (2011) *Service User Experience in Adult Mental Health: Improving the Experience of Care for People Using Adult NHS Mental Health Services. Clinical Guideline 136.* London: National Institute for Health and Clinical Excellence. Available at http://guidance.nice.org.uk/CG136/ NICEGuidance/pdf/English, accessed on 18 January 2015.

Nilforooshan, R., Amin, R. and Warner, J. (2009) 'Ethnicity and outcome of appeal after detention under the Mental Health Act 1983.' *Psychiatric Bulletin 33,* 8, 288–290.

NIMHE (National Institute for Mental Health in England) (2008) *Independent Mental Health Advocacy: Guidance for Commissioners.* Available at http://webarchive. nationalarchives.gov.uk/20130107105354/www.dh.gov.uk/prod_consum_dh/groups/dh_digitalassets/documents/digitalasset/dh_097681.pdf, accessed on 18 January 2015.

NSC NHS Strategic Health Authority (2003) *Independent Inquiry into the Death of David Bennett: An Independent Inquiry set up under HSG (94)27.* Cambridge: NSC NHS Strategic Health Authority.

Nursing and Midwifery Council (2004) *Code of Professional Conduct.* London: Nursing and Midwifery Council.

O'Brien, J. (1987) *Learning from Citizen Advocacy Programs.* Atlanta: Georgia Advocacy Office.

O'Donoghue, B., Lyne, J., Hill, M., Larkin, C., Feeney, L. and O'Callaghan, E. (2010) 'Involuntary admission from the patients' perspective.' *Social Psychiatry and Psychiatric Epidemiology 45,* 6, 631–638.

O'Hagan, M. (2011) *Peer Support in Mental Health and Addictions: A Background Paper.* New Zealand: Kites Trust (self-published).

Ostrom, E. (1996) 'Crossing the great divide: co-production, synergy and development.' *World Development 24,* 6, 1073–1087.

Owiti, J. and Bowers, L. (2010) *A Literature Review: Refusal of Psychotropic Medication in Acute Inpatient Psychiatric Care.* London: Institute of Psychiatry.

PACE (2008) *Project Evaluation: Mental Health Advocacy Project for Advice, Counselling and Education.* London: PACE.

Palmer, D., Nixon, J., Reynolds, S., Panayiotou, A., Palmer, A. and Meyerowitz, R. (2012) 'Getting to know you: reflections on a specialist independent mental health advocacy service for Bexley and Bromley residents in forensic settings.' *Mental Health Review Journal 17,* 1, 5–13.

Papoulias, C., Csipke, E., Rose, D., McKellar, S. and Wykes, T. (2014) 'The psychiatric ward as a therapeutic space: systematic review.' *British Journal of Psychiatry 205,* 3, 171–176.

Parr, H. (2000) 'Interpreting the "hidden social geographies" of mental health: ethnographies of inclusion and exclusion in semi-institutional places.' *Health and Place 6,* 3, 225–237.

Penson, W.J. (2014) 'Psy-science and the colonial relationship in the mental health field.' *Mental Health Review Journal 19,* 3, 176–184.

Perkins, R. and Slade, M. (2012) 'Recovery in England: transforming statutory services?' *International Review of Psychiatry 24,* 1, 29–39.

Perlin, M.L. and Douard, J. (2008) 'Equality, I spoke that word/as if a wedding vow: mental disability law and how we treat marginalized persons.' *New York Law School Law Review 53,* 9.

Perry, A.J.F. (2013) *Inherently Good? A Systematic Review of Qualitative and Quantitative Evidence Regarding Advocacy Intervention Outcomes.* Social Science Research Network. Available at http://dx.doi.org/10.2139/ssrn.2263468, accessed on 29 March 2015.

Piatkowska, O. and Farnill, D. (1992) 'Medication – Compliance or Alliance? A Client Centred Approach to Increasing Adherence.' In D. Kavanagh (ed.) *Schizophrenia: An Overview and Practical Handbook.* London: Chapman and Hall.

Pilgrim, D. (2002) 'The biopsychosocial model in Anglo-American psychiatry: ast, present and future.' *Journal of Mental Health 11,* 585–594.

Pilgrim, D. (2007) 'New "mental health" legislation for England and Wales: some aspects of consensus and conflict.' *Journal of Social Policy 36,* 1, 79–95.

Pilgrim, D. (2008a) 'Reading "happiness": CBT and the Layard thesis.' *European Journal of Psychotherapy and Counselling 10*, 3, 247–260.

Pilgrim, D. (2008b) '"Recovery" and current mental health policy.' *Chronic Illness 4*, 4, 295–304.

Pilgrim, D. (2012a) 'The British welfare state and mental health problems: the continuing relevance of the work of Claus Offe.' *Sociology of Health and Illness 34*, 7, 1070–1084.

Pilgrim, D. (2012b) 'Lessons from the Mental Health Act Commission for England and Wales: the limitations of legalism-plus-safeguards.' *Journal of Social Policy 41*, 1, 61–81.

Pilgrim, D. (2013) 'The failure of diagnostic psychiatry and some prospects of scientific progress offered by critical realism.' *Journal of Critical Realism 12*, 336–358.

Pilgrim, D. (2014a) 'Historical resonances of the DSM-5 dispute: American exceptionalism or Eurocentrism?' *History of the Human Sciences 27*, 2, 97–117.

Pilgrim, D. (2014b) 'The Failure of Modern Psychiatry and Some Prospects of Scientific Progress Offered by Critical Realism.' In E. Speed, J. Moncrieff and M. Rapley (eds) *De-Medicalizing Misery II: Society, Politics and the Mental Health Industry*. Basingstoke: Palgrave Macmillan.

Pilgrim, D. and Ramon, S. (2009) 'English mental health policy under New Labour.' *Policy and Politics 37*, 2, 273–288.

Pilgrim, D. and Rogers, A.E. (2005) 'Psychiatrists as social engineers: a study of an anti-stigma campaign.' *Social Science and Medicine 61*, 12, 2546–2556.

Pinfold, V. (2000) '"Building up safe havens…all around the world": users' experiences of living in the community with mental health problems.' *Health and Place 6*, 3, 201–212.

Plumb, A. (2015) 'UN Convention on the Rights of Persons with Disabilities: Out of the Frying Pan into the Fire? Mental Health Service Users and Survivors Aligning with the Disability Movement.' In H. Spandler, B. Sapey and J. Anderson (eds) *Madness and Distress: Politics of Disablement*. Bristol: Policy Press.

Porter, R. (1990). Mind-Forg'd Manacles. *A History of Madness in England from the Restoration to the Regency*. London: Penguin.

Priebe, S., Katsakou, C., Amos, T., Leese, M. *et al.* (2009) 'Patients' views and readmissions 1 year after involuntary hospitalisation.' *British Journal of Psychiatry 194*, 1, 49–54.

Pringle, R. and Lewis, W. (2014) Personal communication.

Pullen, F. (1995) 'Advocacy: a specialist practitioner role.' *British Journal of Nursing 4*, 275–278.

Purdy, M. (1997) 'Humanist ideology and nurse education. I. Humanist educational theory.' *Nurse Education Today 17*, 3, 192–195.

Quirk, A., Chaplin, R., Lelliott, P. and Seale, C. (2012) 'How pressure is applied in shared decisions about antipsychotic medication: a conversation analytic study of psychiatric outpatient consultations.' *Sociology of Health and Illness 34*, 1, 95–113.

Raboch, J., Kališová, L., Nawka, A., Kitzlerová, E. *et al.* (2010) 'Use of coercive measures during involuntary hospitalization: findings from ten European countries.' *Psychiatric Services 61*, 10, 1012–1017.

Radden, J.H. (2012) 'Recognition rights, mental health consumers and reconstructive cultural semantics.' *Philosophy, Ethics and Humanities in Medicine 7*, 6.

Rai-Atkins, A., Jama, A.A., Wright, N., Scott, V. *et al.* (2002) *Best Practice in Mental Health: Advocacy for African, Caribbean and South Asian Communities*. Bristol: Policy Press.

Raleigh, V.S. and Foot, C. (2010) *Getting the Measure of Quality: Opportunities and Challenges*. London: The King's Fund.

Randall, D. and McKeown, M. (2014) 'Editorial. Failure to care: nursing in a state of liquid modernity?' *Journal of Clinical Nursing 23*, 766–767.

Ravindran, T. and Kelkar-Khambete, A. (2008) 'Gender mainstreaming in health: looking back, looking forward.' *Global Public Health 3*, Suppl. 1, 121–142.

Read, J. and Wallcraft, J. (1994) *Guidelines on the Practice of Advocacy for Mental Health Workers.* London: Unison/Mind.

Read, J., Bentall, R. and Fosse, R. (2014) 'Time to Abandon the Bio-Bio-Bio Model of Psychosis: Exploring the Epigenetic and Psychological Mechanism by Which Adverse Life Events Lead to Psychotic Symptoms.' In E. Speed, J. Moncrieff and M. Rapley (eds) *De-Medicalizing Misery II: Society, Politics and the Mental Health Industry.* Basingstoke: Palgrave Macmillan.

Redley, M., Clare, I., Luke, L. and Holland, A. (2009) 'Mental Capacity Act (England and Wales) 2005: the emergent independent mental capacity advocate (IMCA) service.' *British Journal of Social Work 40*, 1812–1828.

Redley, M., Luke, L., Keeley, H., Clare, I. and Holland, A.J. (2006) *The Evaluation of the Pilot Independent Mental Capacity Advocate (IMCA) Service.* London: Department of Health.

Repper, J. (2011) 'A rights based approach to recovery and social inclusion.' Paper presented at the INTAR conference, 3–4 November, Toronto. Available at www.intar.org/files/INTAR2011-Toronto-JulieRepperARightsBasedApproachToRecoveryandSocial.pdfINTAR conference, accessed on 31 March 2015.

Repper, J. and Perkins, R. (2014) 'The Elephant on the Table.' *Mental Health and Social Inclusion, 18*, 4, doi/abs/10.1108/MHSI-09-2014-0032.

Reville, D. and Church, K. (2012) 'Mad Activism Enters its Fifth Decade: Psychiatric Survivor Organizing in Toronto.' In A. Choudry, J. Hanley and E. Shragge (eds) *Organize! Building from the Local for Social Justice.* Oakland, CA: PM Press.

Richardson, G. (2008) 'Coercion and human rights: a European perspective.' *Journal of Mental Health 17*, 3, 245–254.

Ridley, J. (2014) 'The Experiences of Service Users.' In S. Matthews, P. O'Hare and J. Hemmington (eds) *Approved Mental Health Practice: Essential Themes for Students and Practitioners.* Basingstoke: Palgrave Macmillan.

Ridley, J. and Hunter, S. (2013) 'Subjective experiences of compulsory treatment from a qualitative study of early implementation of the Mental Health (Care and Treatment) (Scotland) Act 2003.' *Health and Social Care in the Community 21*, 5, 509–518.

Ridley, J., McKeown, M., Machin, K., Rosengard, A. *et al.* (2014) *Exploring Family Carer Involvement in Forensic Mental Health Services.* Edinburgh: Support in Mind Scotland.

Ridley, J., Rosengard, A., Hunter, S. and Little, S. (2009) *Experiences of the Early Implementation of the Mental Health (Care and Treatment) (Scotland) Act, 2003: A Cohort Study.* Scottish Government. Available at www.scotland.gov.uk/Publications/2009/05/06155847/0, accessed on 26 January 2015.

Robbins, B.D. (2008) 'What is the good life? Positive psychology and the renaissance of humanistic psychology.' *The Humanistic Psychologist 36*, 2, 96–112.

Roberts, G., Dorkins, E., Wooldridge, J. and Hewis, E. (2008) 'Detained – what's my choice? Part 1: Discussion.' *Advances in Psychiatric Treatment 14*, 3, 172–180.

Robinson, M. (1985) 'Patient advocacy and the nurse: is there a conflict of interest?' *Nursing Forum 22*, 58–63.

Rogers, A. and Pilgrim, D. (1991) '"Pulling down churches": accounting for the British mental health users' movement.' *Sociology of Health and Illness 13*, 2, 129–148.

Rogers, A. and Pilgrim, D. (2014) *A Sociology of Mental Health and Illness*, 5th edition. Maidenhead: Open University Press.

Rogers, A., Pilgrim, D. and Lacey, R. (1993) *Experiencing Psychiatry: Users' Views of Services*. London: Macmillan.

Rogers, C. (1967) *On Becoming a Person: A Therapist's View of Psychotherapy*. London: Constable and Company.

Romme, M. and Escher, S. (1993) *Accepting Voices*. London: Mind Publications.

Rose, D. (2009) 'Survivor Produced Knowledge.' In A. Sweeney, P. Beresford, A. Faulkner, M. Nettle and D. Rose (eds) *This is Survivor Research*. Ross-on-Wye: PCCS Books.

Rose, N. (1986) 'Law, Rights and Psychiatry.' In P. Miller and N. Rose (eds) *The Power of Psychiatry*. Cambridge: Polity Press.

Rose, N. (1990) *Governing the Soul: The Shaping of the Private Self*. London: Routledge.

Rose, S. and Black, B.L. (1985) *Advocacy and Empowerment: Mental Health Care in the Community*. London: Routledge and Kegan Paul.

Rosenberg, C.E. (1975) 'The crisis in psychiatric legitimacy: reflections on psychiatry, medicine and public policy.' *American Psychiatry, Past, Present and Future: Papers Presented on the Occasion of the 200th Anniversary of the Establishment of the First State-Supported Mental Hospital in America*, 135–48.

Rosenhan, D.L. (1973) 'On being sane in insane places.' *Science 179*, 4070, 250–258.

Rosenman, S., Korten, A. and Newman, L. (2000) 'Efficacy of continuing advocacy in involuntary treatment.' *Psychiatric Services 51*, 8, 1029–1033.

Rosenthal, E. and Rubenstein, L.S. (1993) 'International human rights advocacy under the "Principles for the Protection of Persons with Mental Illness".' *International Journal of Law and Psychiatry 16*, 3, 257–300.

Royal College of Psychiatrists (2014) *Accreditation for Inpatient Mental Health Services (AIMS)*. Available at www.rcpsych.ac.uk/workinpsychiatry/qualityimprovement/ qualityandaccreditation/psychiatricwards/aims.aspx, accessed on 18 January 2015.

Ruch, G., Turney, D. and Ward, A. (eds) (2010) *Relationship-Based Social Work: Getting to the Heart of Practice*. London: Jessica Kingsley Publishers.

Rushmer, R. and Hallam, A. (2004) *Mental Health Law in Scotland: Mental Health Law Research Programme. Analysis of Responses to Consultations*. Edinburgh: Scottish Executive.

Russo, J. (2014) 'Mental health service users in research: critical sociological perspectives.' *Disability and Society 29*, 3, 498–500.

Russo, J. and Beresford, P. (2014) 'Between exclusion and colonisation: seeking a place for mad people's knowledge in academia.' *Disability and Society* (ahead-of-print), 1–5. DOI: 10.1080/09687599.2014.957925.

Russo, J. and Rose, D. (2013) '"But what if nobody's going to sit down and have a real conversation with you?" Service user/survivor perspectives on human rights.' *Journal of Public Mental Health 12*, 4, 184–192.

Russo, J. and Wallcraft, J. (2011) 'Resisting Variables: Service User/ Survivor Perspectives on Researching Coercion.' In T.W. Kallert, J.E. Mezzichand and J. Monahan (eds) *Coercive Treatment in Psychiatry: Clinical, Legal and Ethical Aspects*. Chichester, West Sussex/Hoboken, NJ: Wiley-Blackwell.

Ryan, J. with Thomas, F. (1980) *The Politics of Mental Handicap*. Harmondsworth: Penguin.

Ryles, S. (1999) 'A concept analysis of empowerment: its relationship to mental health nursing.' *Journal of Advanced Nursing 29*, 600–607.

Sadd, J. (2014) 'Connecting Psychological Stress and Colonialism.' In J. Weinstein (ed.) *Mental Health: Critical Ideas in Social Work*. Bristol: Policy Press.

Saks, E.R. (2003) 'Involuntary outpatient commitment.' *Psychology, Public Policy and Law 9*, 1–2, 94.

Sang, B. and O'Brien, J. (1984) *Advocacy: The UK and American Experience*. London: King Edward Hospital Fund for London.

Sapey, B. (2013) 'Compounding the trauma: the coercive treatment of voice hearers.' *European Journal of Social Work 16*, 3, 375–390.

Scheff, T. (1966) *Being Mentally Ill: A Sociological Identity*. Chicago: Aldine.

Schopp, R.F. (1993) 'Therapeutic jurisprudence and conflicts among values in mental health law.' *Behavioral Sciences and the Law 11*, 1, 31–45.

SCIE (Social Care Institute for Excellence) (2013) *Coproduction in Social Care: What It Is and How to Do It*. SCIE Guide 51. London: SCIE. Available at www.scie.org.uk/publications/guides/guide51/index.asp, accessed on 2 April 2015.

SCIE (Social Care Institute for Excellence) (2014) *Commissioning Independent Advocacy*. London: SCIE. Available at www.scie.org.uk/care-act-2014/advocacy-services/commissioning-independent-advocacy, accessed on 20 January 2015.

SCIE (Social Care Institute for Excellence) (2015) *IMCA and paid relevant person's representative roles in the Mental Capacity Act Deprivation of Liberty Safeguards*. Available at www.scie.org.uk/publications/guides/guide41/paid.asp, accessed on 7 June 2015.

SCIE/UCLan (Social Care Institute for Excellence/University of Central Lancashire) (2015a) *Independent Mental Health Advocacy (IMHA) Resources*. Available at www.scie.org.uk/independent-mental-health-advocacy/resources-for-users/index.asp, accessed on 29 March 2015.

SCIE/UCLan (Social Care Institute for Excellence/University of Central Lancashire) (2015b). 10 Top tips for commissioners: Commissioning Independent Mental Health Advocacy (IMHA) services in England. Available at www.scie.org.uk/independent-mental-health-advocacy/measuring-effectiveness-and-commissioning/10-top-tips.asp accessed on 18 June 2015.

Scott, B. (2014) 'The broadest shoulders? Disabled people and "welfare reform."' *Concept: The Journal of Contemporary Community Education Practice Theory 5*, 1, 1–10.

Scottish Government (2005) *The New Mental Health Act: What's it all about. A short introduction*. Available at www.gov.scot/Resource/Doc/55971/0015983.pdf accessed on 5 June 2015.

Sectioned (2014a) *Forced Medication: Resistance is Futile*. Available at http://sectioneduk.wordpress.com/2014/03/19/forced-medication, accessed on 21 May 2015.

Sectioned (2014b) *Do You Remember Your First Time?* Available at http://sectioneduk.wordpress.com/2014/11/16/do-you-remember-your-first-time, accessed on 21 May 2015.

Sedgwick, P. (1982) *Psychopolitics*. London: Pluto Press.

Seikkula, J., Alakare, B. and Aaltonen, J. (2011) 'The comprehensive open-dialogue approach in Western Lapland: II. Long-term stability of acute psychosis outcomes in advanced community care.' *Psychosis 3*, 3, 192–204.

Seikkula, J. and Olson, M.E. (2003) 'The open dialogue approach to acute psychosis: its poetics and micropolitics.' *Family Process 42*, 3, 403–418.

Shaughnessy, P. (2001) 'July 9th: day of action. Mad Pride view.' *Asylum: The Magazine for Democratic Psychiatry 13*, 7–8.

Shepherd, G., Boardman, J. and Slade, M. (2007) *Making Recovery a Reality*. London: Sainsbury Centre for Mental Health.

Showalter, E. (1987) *The Female Malady: Women, Madness and English Culture, 1830–1980*. London: Virago.

Sibitz, I., Scheutz, A., Lakeman, R., Schrank, B., Schaffer, M. and Amering, M. (2011) 'Impact of coercive measures on life stories: qualitative study.' *British Journal of Psychiatry 199*, 3, 239–244.

Sign and Mental Health Foundation (undated) *Executive Briefing on Mental Health Services for Deaf and Hard of Hearing People*. Available at www.deafinfo.org.uk/policy/ExecutiveBriefing.pdf, accessed on 9 April 2015.

Silvera, M. and Kapasi, R. (2002) *A Standards Framework for Delivering Effective Health and Social Care Advocacy for Black and Minority Ethnic Londoners*. A Consultancy Partnership Project by SILKCAP and OPM funded by the King's Fund. London: King's Fund.

Slay, J. and Stephens, L. (2013) *Co-Production in Mental Health: A Literature Review*. London: New Economics Foundation.

Smith, D. and David, S. (1975) *Women Look at Psychiatry*. Vancouver: Press Gang Publishers.

Solomon, A. (2012) *Far From the Tree*. New York: NY Books.

Spandler, H. (2006) *Asylum to Action: Paddington Day Hospital, Therapeutic Communities and Beyond*. London: Jessica Kingsley Publishers.

Spandler, H., Anderson, J. and Sapey, B. (eds) (2015) *Distress or Disability? Mental Health and the Politics of Disablement*. Bristol: Policy Press.

Spandler, H. and Calton, T. (2009) 'Psychosis and human rights: conflicts in mental health policy and practice.' *Social Policy and Society 8*, 2, 245–256.

SPN (Social Perspectives Network) (2002) *Start Making Sense…Developing Social Models to Understand and Work with Mental Distress*. Notes from Social Perspectives Network study day, 11 November, SPN paper 3.

Star Wards (2008) *Practical Ideas for Improving the Daily Experiences and Treatment Outcomes of Acute Mental Health In-Patients*. London: Bright. Available at www.starwards.org.uk/category/publications/page/2/ accessed on 5 June 2015.

Stevenson, P. (1989) 'Women in special hospitals.' *OpenMind 41*, 14–16.

Stewart, A. and MacIntyre, G. (2013) *Advocacy: Models and Effectiveness*. IRISS Insights No. 20. Glasgow: IRISS.

Street, C., Anderson, Y., Allan, B., Katz, A., Webb, M. and Roberson, J. (2012) '*It Takes a Lot of Courage': Children and Young People's Experiences of Complaints Procedures in Services for Mental Health and Sexual Health Including Those Provided by GPs*. London: The Children's Commissioner for England.

Stroud, J., Doughty, K. and Banks, L. (2013) *An Exploration of Service User and Practitioner Experiences of Community Treatment Orders*. University of Brighton/NIHR. Available at http://eprints.brighton.ac.uk/12824/1/CTOs-report.pdf, accessed on 8 March 2015.

Stuart, H. (2012) 'United Nations convention on the rights of persons with disabilities: a roadmap for change.' *Current Opinion in Psychiatry 25*, 5, 365–369.

Stylianos, S. and Kehyayan, V. (2012) 'Advocacy: critical component in a comprehensive mental health system.' *American Journal of Orthopsychiatry 82*, 1, 115–120.

Survivors History Group (2012) 'Survivors History Group Takes a Critical Look at Historians.' In M. Barnes and P. Cotterell (eds) *Critical Perspectives on User Involvement*. Bristol: Policy Press.

Sweeney, A., Beresford, P., Faulkner, A., Nettle, M. and Rose, D. (2009) *This is Survivor Research*. Monmouth: PCCS Books.

Szasz, T. (1961) *The Myth of Mental Illness: Foundations of a Theory of Personal Conduct*. New York: Hoeber-Harper.

Szasz, T. (1970) *The Manufacture of Madness*. London: Routledge and Kegan Paul.

Szmukler, G., Daw, R. and Dawson, J. (2010) 'A model law fusing incapacity and mental health legislation.' Special Issue of the *Journal of Mental Health Law*, 11–22.

Teasdale, K. (1999) *Advocacy in Health Care*. London: Blackwell Science.

Tew, J. (2002) 'Going social: championing a holistic model of mental distress within professional education.' *Social Work Education 21*, 2, 143–155.

Thomas, P. (2014) *Psychiatry in Context: Experience, Meaning and Communities*. Monmouth: PCCS Books.

Thomson, G.M. and Downe, S. (2010) 'Changing the future to change the past: women's experiences of a positive birth following a traumatic birth experience.' *Journal of Reproductive and Infant Psychology 28*, 1, 102–112.

Tomes, N. (2006) 'The patient as a policy factor: a historical case study of the consumer/ survivor movement in mental health.' *Health Affairs 25*, 3, 720–729.

Townsley, R. and Laing, A. (2011) *Effective Relationships, Better Outcomes: Mapping the Impact of the Independent Mental Capacity Advocate Service in England* (1 April 2009 to 31 March 2010). London: Social Care Institute for Excellence.

Townsley, R., Marriott, A. and Ward, L. (2009) *Access to Independent Advocacy: An Evidence Review. Report for the Office for Disability Issues*. London: HM Government.

Tudor Hart, J. (1971) 'The inverse care law.' *The Lancet 297*, 405–412.

Tulloch, A.D., Fearon, P. and David, A.S. (2012) 'Timing, prevalence, determinants and outcomes of homelessness among patients admitted to acute psychiatric wards.' *Social Psychiatry and Psychiatric Epidemiology 47*, 7, 1181–1191.

Turner, M. and Beresford, P. (2005) *User Controlled Research: Its Meanings and Potential*. Eastleigh: Involve.

Tyrer, P. (1989) 'Review of "Power in Strange Places: User Empowerment in Mental Health Services".' *Psychiatric Bulletin 13*, 307–308.

Usher, K. and Arthur, D. (1998) 'Process consent: a model for enhancing informed consent in mental health nursing.' *Journal of Advanced Nursing 27*, 692–697.

Ussher, J. (1991) *Women's Madness: Misogyny or Mental Illness?* New York: Harvester Wheatsheaf.

Vaartio, H., Leino-Kilpi, H., Salanterä, S. and Suominen, T. (2006) 'Nursing advocacy: how is it defined by patients and nurses, what does it involve and how is it experienced?' *Scandinavian Journal of Caring Sciences 20*, 3, 282–292.

Valenti, E., Giacco, D., Katasakou, C. and Priebe, S. (2014) 'Which values are important for patients during involuntary treatment? A qualitative study with psychiatric inpatients.' *Journal of Medical Ethics 40*, 12, 832–836.

Vasak, K. (1982) *The International Dimensions of Human Rights* (Vol. 1). Westport, CT: Greenwood Press.

Vige, M. (2009) 'Is independent mental health advocacy working for Black and minority ethnic service users?' *OpenMind 160*, November/ December.

Walker, A. (1989) 'Managing the Package of Care: Implications for the User.' In I. Allen (ed.) *Social Services Departments as Managing Agencies* (PSI Discussion Paper 23). London: Policy Studies Institute.

Wallcraft, J., Amering, M., Freidin, J., Davar, B. *et al.* (2011) 'Partnerships for better mental health worldwide: WPA recommendations on best practices in working with service users and family carers.' *World Psychiatry 10*, 3, 229–236.

Wallcraft, J. and Nettle, M. (2009) 'History, Context and Language.' In J. Wallcraft, B. Schrank and M. Amering (eds) *Handbook of Service User Involvement in Mental Health Research*. Chichester: Wiley and Sons.

Wallcraft, J. with Read, J. and Sweeney, A. (2003) *On Our Own Terms: Users and Survivors of Mental Health Services Working Together for Support and Change.* London: Sainsbury Centre for Mental Health.

Walsh, P. (1985) 'Mental health dilemmas: speaking up for the patient.' *Nursing Times* 81, 24–26.

Ward, L. (ed.) (1998) *Innovations in Advocacy and Empowerment for People with Intellectual Disabilities.* Chorley: Lisieux Hall Publications.

Welsh Government (2011) *Delivering the Independent Mental Health Advocacy Service in Wales.* Available at http://wales.gov.uk/docs/dhss/publications/111222advocacyen. pdf, accessed on 18 January 2015.

Welsh Government, City and Guilds London Institute and Advocacy Training, Consultation and Supervision (2008) *City & Guilds 3610 Level 3 Certificate in Independent Advocacy (IMHA) Learning Support Resource for Unit 306.* Available at Welsh Government (2011) Delivering the Independent Mental Health Advocacy Service in Wales: Guidance for Independent Mental Health Advocacy Providers and Local Health Board Advocacy Service Planners http://gov.wales/docs/dhss/publications/111222advocacyen.pdf accessed on 5 June 2015.

Wessely, S. (2014) *The Real Crisis in Psychiatry is that there isn't Enough of it.* Available at http://theconversation.com/the-real-crisis-in-psychiatry-is-that-there-isnt-enough-of-it-32076, accessed on 18 January 2015.

Westminster Advocacy Service for Senior Residents and Dementia Advocacy Network (2009) *Bringing Dementia Out of the Shadows for BME Elders.* Available at https://lemosandcrane.co.uk/resources/EMDAPReportPDF.pdf, accessed on 25 January 2015.

Wetherell, R. and Wetherell, A. (2008) 'Advocacy: Does it Really Work?' In C. Kaye and M. Howlett (eds) *Mental Health Services Today and Tomorrow: Experiences of Providing and Receiving Care.* Abingdon: Oxford.

White, R.G. and Sashidharan, S.P. (2014) 'Towards a more nuanced global mental health.' *The British Journal of Psychiatry 204,* 6, 415–417.

Whittaker, R. (2002) *Mad in America: Bad Science, Bad Medicine and the Enduring Mistreatment of the Mentally Ill.* New York: Perseus Publishing.

Whittaker, R. (2010) *Anatomy of an Epidemic: Magic Bullets, Psychiatric Drugs and the Astonishing Rise of Mental Illness in America.* New York: Broadway Books.

WHO (World Health Organization) (1958) *The First Ten Years of the World Health Organization.* Geneva: WHO. Available at http://apps.who.int/iris/bitstream/10665/37089/1/a38153.pdf, accessed on 18 January 2015.

WHO (World Health Organization) (2003) *Advocacy for Mental Health.* Geneva: WHO.

WHO (World Health Organization) (2005) *Resource Book on Mental Health: Human Rights and Legislation.* Available at www.who.int/mental_health/policy/resource_book_MHLeg.pdf, accessed on 5 June 2015.

WHO (World Health Organization) Europe (2014) 'How to promote empowerment experiences of mental health service users and carers in Europe? Indicators and good practices.' *4th International WHO–Collaborating Centre for Research and Training in Public Health Congress,* 30–31 January, Lille, France.

Wildeman, S. (2013) 'Protecting rights and building capacities: challenges to global mental health policy in light of the Convention on the Rights of Persons with Disabilities.' *The Journal of Law, Medicine and Ethics 41,* 1, 48–73.

Williams, J. and Stickley, T. (2010) 'Empathy and nurse education.' *Nurse Education Today 30,* 752–755.

Williams, P., Shoultz, B. and Berglas, S. (1984) *We Can Speak for Ourselves: Self-Advocacy by Mentally Handicapped People.* Bloomington, IN: Indiana University Press.

Wilson, A. and Beresford, P. (2000) 'Anti-oppressive practice: emancipation or appropriation?' *British Journal of Social Work 30*, 553–573.

Wilson, M. (2009) *Delivering Race Equality in Mental Health Care: A Review.* London: Department of Health.

Wolfensberger, W. (1972a) *The Principle of Normalization in Human Services.* Toronto, Canada: National Institute on Mental Retardation.

Wolfensberger, W. (1972b) 'Voluntary citizen advocacy in the human services.' *Canada's Mental Health 20*, 2, 14–18.

Wolfensberger, W. (1987/2005) *The New Genocide of Handicapped and Afflicted People*, 3rd (rev) edn. Syracuse, NY: Syracuse University Training Institute for Human Service Planning, Leadership and Change Agentry.

Wood, D. and Pistrang, N. (2004) 'A safe place? Service users' experiences of an acute mental health ward.' *Journal of Community and Applied Social Psychology 14*, 1, 16–28.

Wood, M. and Selwyn, J. (2013) *The Characteristics of Young People Using Independent Advocacy Services.* Bristol: The Hadley Centre, University of Bristol.

Wright, K. (2002) *Reform of the Mental Health Act 1983: The Draft Mental Health Bill. Research Paper 02/80.* House of Commons Library, Social Policy Section. Available at http://researchbriefings.files.parliament.uk/documents/RP02-80/RP02-80.pdf accessed on 5 June 2015.

Wyder, M., Bland, R. and Crompton, D. (2013) 'Personal recovery and involuntary mental health admissions: the importance of control, relationships and hope.' *Scientific Research. Open Access 5*, 3A, 574–581.

Zigmond, A. (1998) 'Medical Incapacity Act.' *Psychiatric Bulletin 22*, 11, 657–658.

Zigmond, A. (2001) 'Reform of the Mental Health Act 1983: the Green Paper.' *Psychiatric Bulletin 25*, 126–128.

Zigmond, A. (2008) 'Changing mental health legislation in the UK.' *Advances in Psychiatric Treatment 14*, 2, 81–83.

Zomorodi, M. and Foley, B. (2009) 'The nature of advocacy vs. paternalism in nursing: clarifying the "thin line".' *Journal of Advanced Nursing 65*, 1746–1752.

Useful Resources

CIE Knowledge review 15: Mtetezi – Developing mental health advocacy with African and Caribbean men Available at www.scie.org.uk/publications/knowledgereviews/kr15.asp

Healthtalk This provides information on a range of health conditions, including mental health, with videos and transcripts of mental health service user experiences. Available at: /www.healthtalk.org

IMROC (Implementing Recovery through Organisational Change) Available at www.imroc.org

Mental Health Law Online Available at www.mentalhealthlaw.co.uk/Mental_Health_Act_2007_Overview

MIND guides to advocacy in mental health Available at www.mind.org.uk/information-support/guides-to-support-and-services/advocacy-in-mental-health/#.VXvyolFFDX4

SCIE/UCLan resources on IMHA services Available at www.scie.org.uk/independent-mental-health-advocacy

At a glance briefing: How to measure the outcomes of IMHA. Available at www.scie.org.uk/independent-mental-health-advocacy/measuring-effectiveness-and-commissioning/impact/index.asp

At a glance briefing: Improving equality of access to IMHA Available at www.scie.org.uk/independent-mental-health-advocacy/improving-equality-of-access/index.asp

At a glance briefing: Quality indicators checklist for providers – what a good service should look like Available at www.scie.org.uk/independent-mental-health-advocacy/measuring-effectiveness-and-commissioning/what-good-imha-service-looks-like/index.asp

At a glance briefing: Top tips for commissioners Available at www.scie.org.uk/independent-mental-health-advocacy/measuring-effectiveness-and-commissioning/10-top-tips.asp

At a glance briefing: Understanding IMHA for mental health staff Available at www.scie.org.uk/independent-mental-health-advocacy/resources-for-staff/understanding/index.asp

At a glance briefing: Understanding IMHA for service users, including easy-read version Available at www.scie.org.uk/independent-mental-health-advocacy/resources-for-users/understanding/index.asp

Improving access to IMHA services through adoption of an open access protocol Available at www.scie.org.uk/independent-mental-health-advocacy/resources-for-staff/improving-access/index.asp

Social Care TV film: For service users Available at www.scie.org.uk/independent-mental-health-advocacy; www.scie.org.uk/independent-mental-health-advocacy/video-player.asp?v=imha-for-people-who-use-services

Social Care TV film: For staff Available at www.scie.org.uk/independent-mental-health-advocacy/video-player.asp?v=imha-for-mental-health-staff

Social Care TV film: Improving equality of access to IMHA. Available at www.scie.org.uk/independent-mental-health-advocacy/video-player.asp?v=imha-improving-equality-of-access

Survivor History Group website Available at http://studymore.org.uk/mhhtim.htm

Subject Index

Author Index

11 Million 227

Aaltonen, J. 111
Action for Advocacy 68,
    182, 183, 189, 190,
    194, 207, 270
Administrative Justice and
    Tribunals Council 139
Advocacy Training,
    Consultation and
    Supervision 204
Ahern, K. 251
Alakare, B. 111
Aldridge, M. 52
Allen, H. 60, 264
Amin, R. 230
Anderson, A. 51, 185
Andreasson, E. 111
Anthony, W. 123, 124
Arthur, D. 248
Ashmore, R. 45
Askey, R. 112
Atkinson, J.M. 136

Bamber, C. 63
Banks, C. 45, 103
Banks, S. 135
Barker, I. 130, 142
Barnes, D. 63, 65, 66, 67, 68,
    86, 90, 130, 131, 165,
    252, 261
Barnes, M. 71, 74
Bartlett, A. 106
Basaglia, F. 58
Bateman, N. 199, 207, 209,
    247, 249, 250, 253
Bauer, A. 18, 193
Beauchamp, T.L. 83
Beeforth, M. 62
Bell, V. 41
Bengtsson-Tops, A. 105
Benjamin, E. 45
Bentall, R. 38, 40, 41, 52
Beresford, P. 29, 49, 50, 51,
    105, 251, 294
Berg-Cross, L. 202
Berglas, S. 23

Bindman, J. 248
Bingley, W. 68–9, 130
Black, B.L. 293–4
Bland, R. 17
Blank, L. 121
Bluglass, R. 68, 80
Boardman, J. 40
Bola, J.R. 52
Bovaird, T. 264
Bowes, A 177
Bowers, L. 115
Bowl, R. 71, 74
Boylan, J. 21, 199, 247, 248,
    294
Bracken, P. 41, 84
Bradley, A. 155
Brady, L. 227, 228
Brandon, A. 55, 57, 86, 136,
    171, 173, 182, 199,
    251, 253
Brandon, D. 55, 57, 59, 171,
    173, 182, 199, 251,
    259, 294
Breggin, P.R. 61
Brett, J. 105
Broadbridge,A. 182, 190
Brooke, J. 207
Brown, G. 140, 143, 280
Bullmore, E. 39
Burstow, B. 50, 51
Busfield, J. 60
Butters, A. 211

Cabinet Office 264
Cadman, A. 59
Caldon, L.J.M. 105
Calton, T. 94, 95
Campbell, P. 55, 56, 57, 62,
    63, 65, 66–7, 72, 177,
    293, 294, 295, 296
Campbell, T. 84
Canvin, K. 106
Care Quality Commission
    (CQC) 27, 89, 96, 103,
    108, 112, 115, 118,
    139, 214, 216, 222,
    240, 274, 283

Carer's Trust 34
Carel, H. 41, 98
Carlsson, H. 127, 130, 131,
    133
Carpenter, M. 94
Carr, S. 237, 240, 282
Carver, N. 130, 131, 133,
    134, 245, 258, 259
Centre for Social Justice 93,
    108, 219
Chamberlin, J. 60, 61, 74
Chesler, P. 60
Children's Commissioner
    for England 227
Church, K. 248
City and Guilds London
    Institute 204
Cleary, M. 248
Cohen, D. 61
Coleman, C. 128
Collins, S. 250
Community Psychiatric
    Nurses Association 59
Conlan, E. 64
Cooke, A. 52, 290
Cooper, L.B. 63
Cornish, F. 177
Cotterell, P. 63
Craig, G. 233, 250, 259
Cresswell, M. 62, 98, 251,
    295
Cromby, J. 41
Crompton, D. 107
Crossley, N. 67
Crowe, M. 47
Cruse, K. 201
Cumbria County Council
    153, 160

Dalrymple, J. 21, 199, 247,
    248, 294
David, S. 60, 121
Davidson, L. 127
Davies, C. 293
Davis, A. 128, 252, 254,
    255, 290
Daw, R. 79, 112